HOW SPORT
AND PHYSICAL ACTIVITY
COULD CONTRIBUTE
TO HUMAN SURVIVAL

Earle F. Zeigler,

Ph.D., LL.D., D.Sc., NAK
The University of Western Ontario
London, Ontario, Canada

2011

Order this book online at www.trafford.com
or email orders@trafford.com

Most Trafford titles are also available at major online book retailers.

Printed in the United States of America.

ISBN: 978-1-4269-8974-2 (sc)
ISBN: 978-1-4269-8975-9 (e)

Trafford rev. 08/05/2011

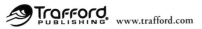 www.trafford.com

North America & international
toll-free: 1 888 232 4444 (USA & Canada)
phone: 250 383 6864 ♦ fax: 812 355 4082

DEDICATION

I have written this book in the hope that those who may read it will realize that the thoughts and ideas expressed here have merit. It is my deep belief that modern, developing civilization is in an increasingly desperate situation.

As the situation relates to human physical activity in exercise, sport, and expressive movement, I wholeheartedly believe that excessive competitive sport has lost its way and overall may be doing more harm than good for those involved and indirectly for the larger populace.

In regard to physical activity education and related educational/recreational sport, I believe we don't understand its potential importance for both "normal" and "special-needs" children and youth. Hence we are missing a golden opportunity to help them live richer, fuller, longer lives...

CONCEPTUAL INDEX

Part		Page
Dedication		3
Conceptual Index		4
Preface		11
I	Introduction: Where in the World Are We?	17
	"The Beginning"	17
	The Use of Sport Down Through the Ages	18
	What *Is* (and *Is Not*) Claimed	19
	A Systemic Change Looms	20
	Solving Such an Enormous Problem	20
	Values Can Be Changed	21
II	An Emerging Postmodern Age	23
	Significant Developments Have "Transformed Our Lives"	24
	The World Has Three Major Trading Blocks	25
	The Impact of Negative Social Forces Has Increased	27
	The Problems of Megalopolis Living Have Not Yet Been Solved	28
	What Character Do We Seek for People?	29
	What Happened to the Original Enlightenment Ideal?	30
	Technology and Improvement of Life	31
	Postmodernism as an Influence	32
III	Was Human Nature Predetermined?	35
	The "Adventure of Civilization"	36
	The Ways Humans Have Acquired Knowledge	37
	Four "Historical Revolutions" in the Development of the World's Communication Capability	39
	Historical Images of Humans' Basic Nature	40
	Seven Rival Theories About Human Nature	42
	Theory #1: Plato–The Rule of the Wise	43
	Theory #2: Christianity–God's Salvation	43
	Theory #3: Marx–Communist Revolution	44

Theory #4: Freud–Psychoanalysis   46
Theory #5: Sartre–Existentialism   48
Theory #6: Skinner–The Conditioning of Behavior   49
Theory #7: Lorenz–Innate Aggression   50
Two Basic Historical Questions   52
The Difficulty of Defining Progress   53
The "Tragic Sense of Life" (Muller)   55
Postscript   56

IV   The Status of Physical Activity Education
and Competitive Sport   58

Introduction   58
Canadian Fitness Level   62
A Terrible Predicament   63
*There is no **profession** of physical education*   64
How Did This Come About Historically   66
We've Got Our Priorities All "Screwed Up"
in Physical Activity Education
and in Competitive Sport   67
Specific Ways That America ("the West?")
Is "Screwing Up" Sport   69
Specific Ways That America ("The West")
Is "Screwing Up" Physical Activity Education   73
How Should Society Solve a Serious Problem?   77
Question 1: Where are we now?
Question 2. Why are we here?
    Citizenry Does Not Comprehend
    the Seriousness of the Issue
    for the Future of Society
Question 3. Where should we want to be?
Question 4. How do we get there?
Question 5. What exactly should we do?
    1. Problem-solving:
    2. Persuasion:
    3. Bargaining:
    4. Politicking:
Children and Youth Need Understanding of,
and Experience With Selected Competencies: 78
1) Correct body mechanics

2) Maintenance of physical fitness (
   cardio-respiratory and strength activities)
3) "Aquatic competence" (how to swim and
   elementary lifesaving)
4) An indoor & an outdoor leisure skill
   (e.g., badminton, tennis, golf)
5) A self-defense activity (major emphasis on defense...)
6) A movement activity (e.g., social dance)

The Public's Conception of 'Physical Education'   78
Concluding Statement   79

V   What Happened With Sport
and Physical Activity Education Historically?   81

Primitive and Preliterate Societies   81
China   81
India   82
Egypt   82
Sumeria (Babylonia and Assyria)   82
Israel   83
Persia   83
Greece   83
   Athenian Greeks   *84*
Rome   84
Visigoths   85
The Early Middle Ages
   (in the West)   86
The Later Middle Ages
   (in the West)   88
Early Modern Period   90
Age of Enlightenment   91
Emerging Nationalism   92
Germany   92
Great Britain   93
The Modern Olympic Games   93
The Twentieth Century   94
The United States of America   94
   The Colonial Period   94
   Early Games, Contests, and Exercise   96
   The 18th Century   96

Early Advocates of "Physical Training"	98
The 19th Century	99
North American Turner	99
Beginning of Organized Sport	101
The Young Men's Christian Association	101
Early Physical Activity in Higher Education	102
An Important Decade for Physical Education	102
The 20th Century	103
Conflicting Educational Philosophies	106
Emergence of the Allied Professions	108
Professional Associations Form Alliance	108
Achieving Some Historical Perspective	109
VI The Sport Hero Phenomenon	111
The Hero in Sport	112
Crepeau on Ruth	112
Insight from History	114
Insight from Sociology	115
Functional Interchanges	115
Insight from Economics	116
Insight from Anthropology	117
Insight from Psychiatry	118
Insight from Philosophy	118
Tiger Woods Was Caught in a Vise: "Socio-Instrumental" Values *and* "Moral" Values Converged to Do Him In!	119
The Occurrence	119
Why Was This Story So Newsworthy?	119
Hard Questions About Present Social Institutions	120
What Happened to the "Enlightenment Ideal"?	121
Challenging the Role of Sport in Society	122
"Socio-Economic", Material Values or "Moral", Non-Material Values?	124
Proposed Tables and Model to Ascertain the Status of Sport Hero	126
Concluding Statement	132

VII   The Olympic Games: A Question of Values   135

Ancient Olympism   135
The (Intended) Goal of Modern Olympism   135
The Problem   136
Social Forces as Value Determinants   138
Use of the Term "Value" in Philosophy   139
Domains of Value Under Axiology   139
An Assessment of the Problem   141
Concluding Statement   143

VIII   Where Should We Want To Be?   144

Status of Physical Activity Education
(including Sport)   144
Questions Parents Might Ask to Improve the Situation   145
What Do You Want for Your Child   145
Are Boys and Girls Rugged Enough?   145
Why Must the Child's Basic Needs Be Met?   145
Why Is Adequate Physical Development Important   146
What Environment Should a Child Have?   146
Why Certain External Pressures Should Be Avoided?   147
Where Do Organized Sports Fit In   148
Why Competitive Sport Offers an Ideal Setting
    for Teaching and Learning?   148
Why Should We Not Introduce Contact/Collision
    Sports Before Maturity?   148
Why Should a Child Not Specialize Unduly at
    an Early Age?   149
Why Should We Offer Youth More in Life
    Than Sport?   150
Why Should We Guarantee the Best Type of
    Sport and Physical Activity Experience to Youth?   150
Under What Circumstances Should We Criticize Those
    Who Sponsor Sports for Youth Too Quickly?   151
What Is a Suggested Formula for the Average Village,
    Town, or City .   151
Let's Ask Ourselves a Few Questions
    About Our Approach to Sport Sponsorship   152
What Is the Challenge of Competitive Sport?   153

IX   Where We Should Be and How Do We Get There?   154

A Call for Professional Reunification   154
Steps That Could Well Be Taken   157
Looking to the Future   159
What to Avoid in the Near Future   162
The Educational Task Ahead:
  Developing a Quality PAE Program
  (including Athletics)   164
    Aims and Objectives   165
    Health and Safety Education (Relationship to...)   167
    Health Services   167
      Health Instruction   168
      Healthful School Living   169
      Physical Education Classification
      or Proficiency Tests   170
    The Basic Required Program   172
      The Conditioning Program   172
      The Sports Instruction Program   172
      The Elective Program   173
    Intramural/Extramural Athletic Competition   173
    Interscholastic or Intercollegiate Athletics   174
    Voluntary Physical Recreation   175
    The Individual or Adaptive Program   176
    Facilities and Equipment   177
    Public Relations   178
    General Administration   179
    Relationship to the Teaching and
      Recreation Professions   180
    Evaluation   181
Major Processes to Achieve
  Desired Objectives and Goals   182
    Problem Solving   182
      1. The Planning Phase   182
      2. Persuasion   183
      3. Bargaining   184
      4. Politicking   185
The Professional Task Ahead   186
The Challenge to the Professional Educator   189

X. Counteracting America's "Western Value" Orientation   191

    Historical Perspective on the "World Situation"   192
    America's Position in the 21st Century   196
    The Impact of Negative Social Forces Has Increased   198
    What Character Do We Seek for People?   199
    What Happened to the Original Enlightenment Ideal?   201
    Future Societal Scenarios (Anderson)   203
    What Kind of A World Do You Want
      for Your Descendents?   204
    Can We Strengthen the Postmodern Influence?   208
    Concluding Statement   211

XI   Sport and Related Physical Activity Education
    in a Postmodern World   212

    Negative Forces Impacting Our Lives   213
    Can Humans Be Both "Judge and Jury"?   214
    America's "Golden Age"?   215
    Five Steps to Problem-Solving   216
    Why Should Competitive Sport Be Unique?   217
    The Sport Hero Phenomenon   218
    Should a Country Support the Olympic Games?   220
    Where Should We Want to Be?   221
    Questions Parents Should Ask   221
    A Final Word   223

References and Bibliography   224

PREFACE

You may think I'm being either pretentious and/or ridiculous by naming this book: *How Sport and Physical Activity Could Contribute to Human Survival.* You could be right about either adjective used, but I intend to do my level best to convince you otherwise. Sport and related physical activity (e.g., work, exercise) have had a long history on earth. Sport, for example, from a simple "throw the ball" beginning has somehow developed to the point where a man can make many millions of dollars just by throwing an inflated pigskin through the air. Or he could be a millionaire many times over–if talented enough!–by persistently keeping a hard-rubber disk from sliding through his legs on ice into a rectangular net that he is "protecting." Further, he could be a billionaire if he hit a golf ball superbly and managed to have a happy family life. However, to this day he must be a male member of the species to earn such a large amount of typically greenish paper known as "currency of the realm" to the cognoscenti.

To earn such large amounts of money, you typically have to do or accomplish something very important in our complex society. Even so, how could such seemingly simple maneuvers with–say–an object of one type or another be worth so much to the performer? The answer is simple or complex depending upon how or where it is done–and under what circumstances. This is the interesting, perhaps ridiculous, aspect of the development of a game or sport generally that has grown so disproportionately important during the 20th century of humankind's life on a speck in the universe known as Earth. Parenthetically, Earth is located in an infinite galaxy of astral bodies known colloquially as the universe. Or is it multi-verse?

To bring my narrative "back to earth," I will now "begin at the beginning" by telling you how I decided to try to affirm (to me first!) these seemingly evident truths to you, the reader. I thought the world (Earth!) would be in better shape by the time I died (ha!), but it appears to be in a "worse mess" than when I started more than 92 years ago. Disturbingly, also, the news of "fresh disasters" is arriving faster and with greater detail because of improved communication globally. And such news is increasingly more of "a mess" daily no matter how or from what direction you look at it! Natural disasters simply occur, but the "impending disaster" I am fearing has been brought about by a creature known as "man" or "woman" (mostly man!).

O.K. So let us assume that impending disaster looms. What about it? And where do sport and related physical activity (exercise!) fit into this discussion? Since the evolution of our species on land began, human physical activity in sport, exercise, and physical recreation has become an increasingly important and vital aspect of the life of those "humans" who are now in "essential control" of the planet.

My chosen task in this book is to show that sport and related physical activity assumed greater or lesser importance starting with primitive societies and continued in later societies on down to the present day. As a social force impacting society generally, and also as a vital concern for those desiring to employ it professionally in a variety of ways within society, such activity was used to help people of all ages in a variety of ways as they lived out their lives.

However, as is the case with so many facets of life on Earth, such involvement can be used beneficially or misused to the subsequent improvement or detriment of humankind. It is my thesis that we are using it well in some ways, *but that we are also abusing it badly in others!* In the case of competitive sport, I believe we have gradually abused it (i.e., perhaps reaching a stage where could well be doing more harm than good with it). Conversely, in the case of related physical activity (i.e., regular exercise or "physical activity education") in the developed world, I believe humans are too often "abusing it by first not understanding it and then by not using it more intelligently"! (And, ironically, in the "undeveloped world," people often get *too much* "exercise" just to stay alive!)

As I see it, with sport we are using it, or people are "using us". but not to its best advantage. In the case of exercise, we are using it insufficiently—and therefore not to its best advantage either. How this has happened since earliest times is the task I have chosen for myself to explain in this book.

Please understand this, however: I don't for a moment argue here that (1) the proper use of sporting activities throughout the earth's affairs could be a panacea for all of the world's ills, the elixir that would create a heretofore unknown era of good will and peace worldwide. I do believe that, wisely employed, it could enrich lives "healthwise" and recreationally for many more millions than it is doing presently. In addition, I do assert (2) that *the wise use of exercise and sound health practices throughout people's entire lives would indubitably go a long way toward keeping people happier and healthier in longer lives extended because of this type of life practice.*

What I am arguing is that, employed properly and correctly, sport and related physical activity—*as one of a number of vital social forces (e.g., nationalism, ecology)*—could contribute to the improvement of the current situation enormously. Moreover, I believe that the active use of competitive sport worldwide to promote what have been called ***moral***, non-material values, traits or attributes, as opposed to so-called ***socio-instrumental,*** *material* values, would create a social force of such strength and power that humankind might be saved from the social and physical devastation looming ahead. At the very least, I believe such active promotion would delay to a considerable degree the onset of what promises to be a most untenable societal situation.)

Such an "untenable societal scenario" has been described vividly by Walter Truett Anderson in the essay "Futures of the Self," taken from *The Future of the Self: Inventing the Postmodern Person* (1997). He sketched four different scenarios as postulations for the future of earthlings in this ongoing adventure of civilization. Anderson's "One World, Many Universes" version is the most likely to occur. This is a scenario characterized by high economic growth, steadily increasing technological progress, and globalization combined with high psychological development. Such psychological maturity, he predicts, will be possible for a certain segment of the world's population because "active life spans will be gradually lengthened through various advances in health maintenance and medicine" (pp. 251-253)

Nevertheless, a problem has developed with this dream of individual achievement of inalienable rights and privileges. In a world where globalization and economic "progress" seemingly must be rejected because of catastrophic environmental concerns or "demands," the bold-future image could well "be replaced by a post-modern self; off-centered, multidimensional, and changeable" (p. 50).

The systemic-change force mentioned above—that is shaping the future. This all-powerful force may well exceed the Earth's ability to cope. As gratifying as such factors as "globalization along with economic growth" and "psychological development" may seem to the folks in a coming "One-World, Many Universes" scenario, there is a flip side to this prognosis. Anderson identifies this image as "The Dysfunctional Family" scenario. All of these benefits of so-called progress are highly expensive and available now only to relatively few of the six billion plus people on earth. Anderson foresees this as "a world of modern people happily doing their thing; of modern people still obsessed with progress, economic gain, and organizational bigness; and of postmodern people being trampled and getting angry" [italics added] (p. 51). As people get angrier, present-day terrorism in North America could seem like child's play.

Hence, the charge I have given myself is to make the case that civilization is steadily giving evidence that (1) the social phenomenon known as competitive sport is largely being used incorrectly, and (2) the social phenomenon known as planned physical activity education (and related health education) is being employed insufficiently and inadequately. Both of these activities promoted one way or another could combine to make a social force that used properly could go a long way to the creation of a better, more peaceful world. ***Presently I believe that the relationship between these two aspects of a potentially most powerful social force is "out of joint." It must be rectified!***

Exactly how to tackle this enormous problem (i.e., bring the "two aspects of this powerful social force of human physical movement" back "in joint" is the tremendously complex task that faces a world that doesn't appear to recognize the depth and intensity of the debilitating problem that has emerged. First, it would be necessary to "enlighten" a substantive majority of the world's population, and then the actual "enlightenment" would have to result in the implementation of these two premises in daily practice. Hence it appears that my task is to first try to explain how ***"it"*** happened (i.e., this "disjointedness"). Then, when I have delineated the problematic situation as clearly as possible, I will try to explain exactly what would have to happen so that the two aspects of this powerful social force can be balanced in a way that will ***help*** humankind survive–and not continue to ***hinder***–in the years ahead.

Succinctly, then, I will seek to seek to trace the problem historically. I will describe briefly the social forces that affect society, and I will explain how the social force of ***values*** influences all other values. As I get to the 20th century, I will explain why America, despite its' professed good intentions and actions–actions often executed for better or worse!–shares a good portion of the blame for humankind's dilemma.

Next I will single out sport and physical activity education portraying how it (together!) has become one of these contradictory social forces, one that is increased in influence down to the present day. In the process I will explain how completed research is telling us that sport is being used ever more to promote what have been designated as "socio-instrumental", material values rather than to promote the ultimately more desirable "moral", non-material value development.

> (Note: The terminology immediately above here is confusing as it seeks to convey specified meanings.)

As I proceed, I will try to explain precisely what changes would have to occur in sport to convince people as to the direction we *must* take. Then I will describe what type of physical activity education seems necessary and most desirable for the very large majority of people who are either "under-exercised" or "over-exercised" (in each case because of their imposed or elected lifestyle).

Admittedly, all of this sounds like an impossible task, and to you the reader it may not make sense. To me, however, it does seem possible, even plausible, if we work collectively to promote the appropriate level of physical activity for people of all ages throughout the world.

You may ask how this could be possible if the social force of *values* is so dominant thereby influencing all other social forces "beneath" it on the prevailing scale of values. The answer is that values are *not*—*should not be*!—rigid and inflexible in all regards. They should be human-made! As we understand what works for the "desired good" in our daily lives for the betterment of humankind, these more beneficial, more desirable values should be implemented!

Hence, if people can be convinced to promote the "right kind" of competitive sport and the right kind and amount of physical activity (exercise!), this type of "adjustment" could conceivably bring about certain *overall* change in the world's prevailing value structure.

I conclude by asking: "What have we to lose, if we don't do everything possible to bring these two related aspects of a growing and/or declining social force into an acceptable alignment?" To this query, I reply simply: "In conjunction with other strong social forces, the answer to this question is *everything*!"

Earle F. Zeigler

PART I
Introduction:

You may think I'm being either pretentious and/or ridiculous by naming this book: *How Sport Could Contribute to Human Survival.* Many others might agree with you about either or both adjectives used, but I intend to do my level best to convince you otherwise. Sport and other physical activity (e.g., work, exercise) have had a long history on earth. Sport, for example, from a very humble beginning has somehow developed to the point where a man can make many millions of dollars just by throwing joined and inflated parts of a pigskin through the air. Or he could be a millionaire many times over–if talented enough!–by persistently keeping a hard-rubber disk from sliding through his legs on ice into a rectangular net that he is "protecting." However, to this day he must be a male member of the species to earn such a large amount of typically greenish paper known as "currency of the realm" to the cognoscenti.

To earn such large amounts of money, you typically have to do or accomplish something very important in our complex society. Even so, how could such seemingly simple maneuvers with–say–an object of one type or another be worth so much to the performer? (Of course, this only happens if there is an accompanying arena seating many thousands of people who pay often hard-earned money to sit on the "fannies" and watch someone else get exercise...) The answer is simple or complex depending upon how or where it is done–and under what circumstances. This is the interesting, perhaps ridiculous, aspect of the development of a activity called sport generally worldwide that grew so disproportionately important during the 20th century of humankind's life on a speck in the universe known as Earth. In addition, as it happens, Earth is located in an infinite galaxy of astral bodies known colloquially as "the universe." Or is it "multi-verse?"

"The Beginning"

To bring my narrative "back to earth," I will now "begin at the beginning" by telling you why I decided to try to affirm (to me first!) this evident truth to you, the reader. In the early years of my life I thought the world (Earth!) would be in better shape by the time I died (ha!). It appears now to be in a "worse mess" in many ways than when I started breathing in it more than 90 years ago. Disturbingly, also, today the news of "fresh disasters" is arriving faster and with greater detail because of improved communication globally. And such news is increasingly of a nature to be described as "a mess" daily–no matter how or from what direction you look at it! Natural disasters simply occur, but the "impending or looming disaster" I am fearing has been brought about by a creature known as "man" or "woman" (mostly male, I confess!).

O.K. So let us assume that impending disaster looms. What about it? And where do sport and related physical activity (exercise!) fit into this discussion? Somehow, since the evolution of our species on land began, human physical activity in sport, exercise, and physical recreation has become an increasingly important and vital aspect of the life of those organisms ("humans"!) who are now in "essential control" of the planet as far as they can tell.

The Use of Sport Down Through the Ages

My chosen task in this book is to point out that sport and related physical activity in its development has assumed greater or lesser importance starting with primitive societies and continued in later societies on down to the present day. Such activity, as a social force impacting society generally, and also as a vital concern for those desiring to employ it professionally in a variety of ways within society, has been used to help people of all ages in a variety of ways as they lived out their lives.

However, as is the case with so many facets of life on Earth, such involvement can be used beneficially or misused to the subsequent improvement or detriment of humankind. Here I argue strenuously that we are using it well in some ways, *but that we are also abusing it badly in others!* In the case of competitive sport, I believe we have gradually abused it (i.e., perhaps reaching a stage where could well be doing more harm than good with it). Conversely, in the case of related physical activity (i.e., regular exercise or "physical activity education") in the developed world, I believe humans are too often "abusing it by first not understanding it and then by not using it more intelligently"! (Oddly, in the "undeveloped world," people often get *too much* exercise (i.e., work!) just to stay alive and cope with daily problems!)

With sport, we are using it, or people are "using it", but not to its best advantage. In the case of exercise, we are using it insufficiently—and therefore not to its best advantage either. How this has happened since earliest times is the task I have chosen for myself to explain in this book.

What *Is* (and *Is Not*) Claimed...

Please understand this, however: I don't for a moment argue that (1) the proper use of sporting activities throughout the earth's affairs could be a panacea for *all* of the world's ills, the elixir that would create a heretofore unknown era of good will and peace worldwide. I do believe that, wisely employed, it could enrich lives "health–wise" and recreationally for many more millions than it is doing presently. *Conversely, I do assert (2) that the wise use of exercise and sound health practices throughout people's entire lives would indubitably go a long way toward keeping people happier and healthier in longer lives extended because of this type of life practice.*

What I am arguing is that, employed properly and correctly, sport and related physical activity–*as one of a number of vital social forces (e.g., healthy patriotism, sound ecological practice)*–could contribute to the improvement of the current situation enormously. Moreover, I believe that the active use of competitive sport worldwide to promote what have been called *moral* (or *non-material*) values, traits or attributes, as opposed to so-called *socio-instrumental* (or *material*) values, would create a social force of such strength and power that humankind might be saved from the social and physical devastation looming ahead. *At the very least, I believe such active promotion would delay to a considerable degree the onset of what promises to be before too long to be a an untenable societal situation.)*

Such an "untenable societal scenario" has been described vividly by Walter Truett Anderson in the essay "Futures of the Self," taken from *The Future of the Self: Inventing the Postmodern Person* (1997). Anderson sketched four different scenarios as postulations for the future of earthlings in this ongoing adventure of civilization. To me it seems that Anderson's "One World, Many Universes" version is the most likely to occur. This is a scenario characterized by (1) high economic growth, (2) steadily increasing technological progress, and (3) globalization combined with high psychological development. Such psychological maturity, he predicts, will be possible for a certain segment of the world's population because "active life spans will be gradually lengthened through various advances in health maintenance and medicine" (pp. 251-253)

A Systemic Change Forces Looms...

Nevertheless, a problem has developed with this dream of individual achievement of inalienable rights and privileges. In a world where now globalization and economic "progress" seemingly must be rejected because of catastrophic environmental concerns or "demands," Anderson's "bold-future image" could well "be replaced by a post-modern self; de–centered, multidimensional, and changeable" (p. 50).

The systemic-change force mentioned above- that will shape the future–this all-powerful force– may well exceed the Earth's ability to cope. As gratifying as such factors as "globalization along with economic growth" and "psychological development" may seem to the folks in a coming "One-World, Many Universes" scenario, there is a flip side to this prognosis. Anderson identifies this image as "The Dysfunctional Family" scenario. All of these benefits of so-called progress are highly expensive and available now only to relatively few of the soon-to-be seven billion people on earth. Anderson foresees this as "a world of modern people happily doing their thing; of modern people still obsessed with progress, economic gain, and organizational bigness; and of postmodern people being trampled and getting angry" (p. 51). And, as more and more people get angrier worldwide, present-day terrorism in North America and elsewhere may well seem like child's play.

Hence, the charge I have given myself in this book is to make the case that civilization is steadily giving evidence that (1) the social phenomenon known as competitive sport is largely being used incorrectly, and (2) the social phenomenon known as planned, daily physical activity education (and related health education) is being employed insufficiently and inadequately. Both of these activities promoted one way or another could combine–if used properly!–to make a social force that could go a long way to the creation of a better, more peaceful world. *Presently I believe that the relationship between these two aspects of a potentially most powerful social force is "out of joint." It must be rectified if we hope for a better future for humankind!*

Solving Such An Enormous Problems

Exactly how to tackle this enormous problem (i.e., bring the two aspects of this powerful social force back "in joint") is the tremendously complex task that faces a world that doesn't appear to recognize the depth and intensity of the problem–or in many cases that a problem even exists!. First, it would be necessary to "enlighten" a substantive majority of the world's population, and then such actual "enlightenment" would have to result in the implementation of these two premises in daily practice. Hence it appears that my task is to first try to explain how "*it*" happened (i.e., this "disjointedness"). Then, when I have delineated the problematic situation as clearly as possible, I will try to explain exactly what would have to happen so that the two aspects of this powerful social force can be balanced in a way that will *help* humankind survive—and not continue to *hinder*—in the years ahead.

Succinctly, then, I will seek to seek to trace the problem historically. I will describe briefly the social forces that affect society, and I will explain how the social force of *values* influences all other values. As I get to the 20th century, I will explain why America, despite its professed good intentions and actions—and often executed ones!—shares a good portion of the blame for humankind's dilemma.

Next I will single out sport and physical activity education portraying how it (together!) has become one of these social forces, one that is increased in influence down to the present day. In the process I will explain how completed research is telling us that sport is being used ever more to promote what have been designated as "socio-instrumental" or material values than to promote so-called "moral" or non-material value development. (Note: The terminology here is a bit confusing as it seeks to convey specified meanings.)

In conclusion, I will try to explain precisely what changes would have to occur in sport to convince people as to the direction we *must* take. Finally I will describe what type of physical activity education seems necessary and most desirable for the very large majority of people who are either "under-exercised" or "over-exercised" (in each case because of their imposed or elected lifestyle).

Values Can Be Changed

Admittedly, all of this sounds like an impossible task. To me, however, it does seem possible, even plausible, if we work collectively to promote the appropriate level and type of physical activity for people of all ages throughout the world.

You may ask how this could be possible if the social force of *values* is so dominant thereby influencing all other social forces "beneath" it on the prevailing scale of values. The answer is that our values are *not*–**should not be**!–rigid and inflexible in all regards. *They should be human-made!* As we understand what works for the "desired good" in our daily lives for the betterment of humankind, these values should be implemented!

Hence, if people can be convinced to promote the "right kind" of competitive sport and the "right kind" of physical activity (exercise!), this type of "adjustment" could conceivably bring about some **overall** change in the world's prevailing value structure governing this aspect of human life.

I conclude by asking: "What have we to lose, if we don't do everything possible to bring these two related aspects of a growing social force into an acceptable alignment?" To this question, I reply simply: "In conjunction with other strong social forces operative, **everything**!"

PART II
An Emerging Postmodern Age

Most North Americans do not fully comprehend that their unique position in the history of the world's development will in all probability change radically in the 21st century. For that matter. the years ahead are really going to be difficult ones for all of the world's citizens. The United States, as the one major nuclear power, has assumed the ongoing, massive problem of maintaining large-scale peace. Of course, a variety of countries, both large and small, may or may not have nuclear arms capability as well. That is what is so worrisome.

Additionally, all of the world will be having increasingly severe ecological problems, not to mention the ebbs and flows of an energy crisis. Generally, also, there is a worldwide nutritional problem, as well as an ongoing situation where the rising expectations of the underdeveloped nations, including their staggering debt (and ours!), will somehow have to be met. These are just a few of the major concerns looming on the horizon.

Indeed, although it is seemingly truer of the United States than Canada, history is going against Americans in several ways. This means that their previous optimism must be tempered to shake them loose from delusions they have acquired For example, despite the presence of the United Nations, the United States has persisted in envisioning itself—as the world superpower—as almost being endowed by the Creator to make all crucial political decisions. Such decisions, often to act unilaterally with the hoped-for, but belated sanction of the United Nations, have resulted in United States-led incursions in the Middle East in Iraq and Afghanistan and into Somalia for very different reasons. And there are other similar situations that are now history (e.g., Cuba, Afghanistan, the former Yugoslavia, Rwanda, Sudan, Haiti, respectively, not to mention other suspected incursions).

Nevertheless, there is reason to expect selected American retrenchment brought on by its excessive world involvement and enormous debt. Of course, any such retrenchment would inevitably lead to a decline in the economic and military influence of the United States. But who can argue logically that the present uneasy balance of power is a healthy situation looking to the future? Norman Cousins appeared to have sounded just the right note more than a generation ago when he stated that "the most important factor in the complex equation of the future is the way the human mind responds to crisis"

(1974, 6-7). The world culture as we know it must respond adequately to the many challenges with which it is being confronted. The societies and nations must individually and collectively respond positively, intelligently, and strongly if humanity as we have known it is to survive.

Significant Developments Have "Transformed Our Lives"

In this brief discussion of national and international developments, with an eye to achieving some historical perspective on the subject, we should also keep in mind the specific developments in the last quarter of the 20th century. For example, Naisbitt (1982) outlined the "ten new directions that are transforming our lives," as well as the "megatrends" insofar as women's evolving role in societal structure (Aburdene & Naisbitt, 1992). Here I am referring to:

(1) the concepts of the information society and the Internet,
(2) "high tech/high touch,"
(3) the shift to world economy,
(4) the need to shift to long-term thinking in regard to ecology,
(5) the move toward organizational decentralization,
(6) the trend toward self-help,
(7) the ongoing discussion of the wisdom of participatory democracy as opposed to representative democracy,
(8) a shift toward networking,
(9) a reconsideration of the "north-south" orientation, and
(10) the viewing of decisions as "multiple option" instead of "either/or."

Add to this the ever-increasing, lifelong involvement of women in the workplace, politics, sports, organized religion, and social activism, Now we begin to understand that a new world order has descended upon us as we begin the 21st century.

Moving ahead in time slightly beyond Naisbitt's first set of *Megatrends*, a second list of 10 issues facing political leaders was highlighted as "Ten events

24

that shook the world between 1984 and 1994" (*Utne Reader*, 1994, pp. 58-74). Consider the following:

(1) the fall of communism and the continuing rise of nationalism,

(2) the environmental crisis and the Green movement,

(3) the AIDS epidemic and the "gay response,"

(4) continuing wars and the peace movement,

(5) the gender war,

(6) religion and racial tension,

(7) the concept of "West meets East" and resultant implications,

(8) the "Baby Boomers" came of age and "Generation X" has started to worry and complain because of declining expectation levels,

(9) the whole idea of globalism and international markets, and

(10) the computer revolution and the specter of Internet.

The World Has Three Major Trading Blocks

Concurrent with the above developments, to help cope with such change the world's "economic manageability" may have been helped by its division into three major trading blocs: (1) the Pacific Rim dominated by Japan, (2) the European Community very heavily influenced by Germany, and (3) North America dominated by the United States of America. While this appears to be true to some observers, interestingly perhaps something even more fundamental has occurred. Succinctly put, world politics seems to be "entering a new phase in which the fundamental source of conflict will be neither ideological nor economic." In the place of these, Samuel P. Huntington, of Harvard's Institute for Strategic Studies, believes that now the major conflicts in the world will actually be clashes between different groups of civilizations espousing fundamentally different cultures (*The New York Times*, June 6, 1993, E19).

These clashes, Huntington states, represent a distinct shift away from viewing the world as being composed of first, second, and third worlds as was the case during the cold war. Thus, Huntington is arguing that in the 21st century the world will return to a pattern of development evident several hundred years ago in which civilizations will actually rise and fall. (Interestingly, this is exactly what was postulated by the late Arnold Toynbee in his earlier famous theory of history development.)

Thus, internationally, with the dissolution of the Union of Soviet Socialist Republics (USSR), Russia and the remaining communist regimes are being severely challenged as they seek to convert to more of a capitalistic economic system. Additionally, a number of other multinational countries have either broken up, or are showing signs of potential breakups (e.g., Yugoslavia, China, Canada). Further, the evidence points to the strong possibility that the developing nations are becoming ever poorer and more destitute with burgeoning populations and widespread starvation setting in.

Further, Western Europe is facing a demographic time bomb even more than the United States because of the influx of refugees from African and Islamic countries, not to mention refugees from countries of the former Soviet Union. It appears further that the European Community will be inclined to appease Islam's demands. However, the multinational nature of the European Community will tend to bring on economic protectionism to insulate its economy against the rising costs of prevailing socialist legislation.

Still further, there is some evidence that Radical Islam, along with Communist China, may well become increasingly aggressive toward the Western culture of Europe and North America. At present, Islam gives evidence of replacing Marxism as the world's main ideology of confrontation. For example, Islam is dedicated to regaining control of Jerusalem and to force Israel to give up control of land occupied earlier to provide a buffer zone against Arab aggressors. (Also, China has been arming certain Arab nations. But how can we be too critical in this regard when we recall that the U.S.A. has also armed selected countries in the past [and present?] when such support was deemed in its interest?)

As Hong Kong is absorbed into Communist China, further political problems seem inevitable in the Far East as well. Although North Korea is facing agricultural problems, there is the possibility (probability?) of the building of nuclear bombs there. (Further, there is the ever-present fear worldwide that small nations and terrorists will somehow get nuclear weapons too.) A growing Japanese assertiveness in Asian and world affairs also seems inevitable because of its typically very strong financial position. Yet the flow of foreign capital from Japan into North America has slowed down somewhat because Japan is being confronted with its own financial crisis caused by inflated real estate and market values. There would obviously be a strong reaction to any fall in living standards in this tightly knit society. Interestingly, still further, the famed Japanese work ethic has become somewhat tarnished by the growing attraction of leisure opportunities.

The situation in Africa has become increasingly grim because the countries south of the Sahara Desert (that is, the dividing line between black Africa and the Arab world) experienced extremely bad economic performance in the past two decades). This social influence has brought to a halt much of the continental effort leading to political liberalization while at the same time exacerbating traditional ethnic rivalries. This economic problem has accordingly forced governmental cutbacks in many of the countries because of the pressures brought to bear by the financial institutions of the Western world that have been underwriting much of the development. The poor are therefore getting poorer, and health (AIDs!) and education standards have in many instances deteriorated even lower than they were previously.

The Impact of Negative Social Forces Has Increased

Now, shifting the focus of this discussion from the problems of an unsettled "Global Village" back to the problem of "living the good life" in the 21st century in North America, we are finding that the human recreational experience will have to be earned typically within a society whose very structure has been modified. For example, (1) the concept of the traditional family structure has been strongly challenged by a variety of social forces (e.g., economics, divorce rate); (2) many single people are finding that they must work longer hours; and (3) many families need more than one breadwinner just to make ends meet. Also, the idea of a steady surplus economy may have vanished, temporarily it is hoped, in the presence of a substantive drive to reduce a budgetary deficit by introducing major cutbacks in so-called nonessentials.

The Problems of Megalopolis Living
Have Not Yet Been Solved

Additionally, many of the same problems of megalopolis living described as early as the 1960s still prevail and are even increasing (e.g., declining infrastructure, rising crime rates, transportation gridlocks, overcrowded schools). Interestingly, in that same year of 1967, Prime Minister Lester Pearson asked Canadians to improve "the quality of Canadian life" as Canada celebrated her 100th anniversary as a confederation. And still today, despite all of Canada's current identity problems, she can take some pride in the fact that Canada has on occasion been proclaimed as the best place on earth to live (with the United States not very far behind). Nevertheless, we can't escape the fact that the work week is not getting shorter and shorter. Also, Michael's prediction about four different types of leisure class still seems a distant dream for the large majority of people.

Further, the situation has developed in such a way that the presently maturing generation, so-called Generation X, is finding that fewer good-paying jobs are available and the average annual income is declining (especially if we keep a steadily rising cost of living in mind). What caused this to happen? This is not a simple question to answer. For one thing, despite the rosy picture envisioned a generation ago, one in which we were supposedly entering a new stage for humankind, we are unable today to cope adequately with the multitude of problems that have developed. This situation is true whether inner city, suburbia, exurbia, or small-town living are concerned. Transportation jams and gridlock, for example, are occurring daily as public transportation struggles to meet rising demand for economical transport within the framework of developing megalopolises.

Certainly, megalopolis living trends have not abated and will probably not do so in the predictable future. More and more families, where that unit is still present, need two breadwinners just to survive. Interest rates, although minor cuts are made when economic slowdowns occur, remain quite high. This discourages many people from home ownership. Pollution of air and water continues despite efforts of many to change the present course of development. High-wage industries seem to be "heading south" in search of places where lower wages can be paid. Also, all sorts of crime are still present in our society, a goodly portion of it seemingly brought about by unemployment and rising debt at all levels from the individual to the federal government. The rise in youth crime is especially disturbing. In this respect, it is fortunate in North America that municipal, private-agency, and public recreation has received continuing financial support from the increasingly burdened taxpayer. Even here, however, there has been a definite trend toward user fees for many services.

What Character Do We Seek for People?

Still further, functioning in a world that is steadily becoming a "Global Village," we need to think more seriously than ever before about the character and traits for which we should seek to develop in people. The so-called developed nations can only continue to lead or strive for the proverbial good life if children and young people develop the right attitudes (psychologically speaking) toward (1) education, (2) work, (3) (use of leisure), (4) participation in government, (5) various types of consumption, and (6) concern for world stability and peace. Make no mistake about it. If we truly desire "the good life," education for the creative and constructive use of leisure—as a significant part of ongoing general education—should have a unique role to play from here on into the indeterminate future.

What are called the Old World countries all seem to have a "character." It is almost something that they take for granted. However, it is questionable whether there is anything that can be called a character in North America (i.e., in the United States, in Canada). Americans were thought earlier to be heterogeneous and individualistic as a people, as opposed to Canadians. But the Canadian culture—whatever that may be today!—has changed quite a bit in recent decades toward multiculturalism — not to mention French-speaking Quebec, of course—as people arrived from many different lands. (Of course, Canada was founded by two distinct cultures, the English and the French.)

Shortly after the middle of the twentieth century, Commager (1966), the noted historian, enumerated what he believed were some common denominators in American (i.e., U.S.) character. These, he said, were (1) carelessness; (2) openhandedness, generosity, and hospitality; (3) self-indulgence; (4) sentimentality, and even romanticism; (5) gregariousness; (6) materialism; (7) confidence and self-confidence; (8) complacency, bordering occasionally on arrogance; (9) cultivation of the competitive spirit; (10) indifference to, and exasperation with laws, rules, and regulations; (11) equalitarianism; and (12) resourcefulness (pp. 246-254).

What about Canadian character as opposed to what Commager stated above? To help us in this regard, a generation ago, Lipset (1973) made a perceptive comparison between the two countries. After stating that they probably resemble each other more than any other two countries in the world, he asserted that there seemed to be a rather "consistent pattern of differences between them" (p. 4). He found that certain "special differences" did exist and may be singled out as follows:

Varying origins in their political systems and national identities, varying religious traditions, and varying frontier experiences. In general terms, the value orientations of Canada stem from a counterrevolutionary past, a need to differentiate itself from the United States, the influence of Monarchical institutions, a dominant Anglican religious tradition, and a less individualistic and more governmentally controlled expansion of the Canadian than of the American frontier (p. 5).

What Happened to the Original Enlightenment Ideal?

The achievement of "the good life" for a majority of citizens in the developed nations, a good life that involves a creative and constructive use of leisure as a key part of general education, necessarily implies that a certain type of progress has been made in society. However, we should understand that the chief criterion of progress has undergone a subtle but decisive change since the founding of the United States republic, for example. This development has had a definite influence on Canada and Mexico as well. Such change has been at once a cause and a reflection of the current disenchantment of some with technology. Recall that the late 18th century was a time of political revolution when monarchies, aristocracies, and the ecclesiastical structure were being challenged on a number of fronts in the Western world. Also, the factory system was undergoing significant change at that time. Such industrial development with its greatly improved machinery "coincided with the formulation and diffusion of the modern Enlightenment idea of history as a record of progress..." (Marx, 1990, p. 5).

Thus, this "new scientific knowledge and accompanying technological power was expected to make possible and practical a comprehensive improvement in all of the conditions of life— social, political, moral, and intellectual as well as material." This idea did indeed slowly take hold and eventually "became the fulcrum of the dominant American world view" (Marx, p. 5). By 1850, however, with the rapid growth of the United States especially, the idea of progress was already being dissociated from the Enlightenment vision of political and social liberation.

Technology and Improvement of Life

By the turn of the twentieth century, "the technocratic idea of progress [had become] a belief in the sufficiency of scientific and technological innovation as the basis for general progress" (Marx, p. 9). This came to mean that if scientific-based technologies were permitted to develop in an unconstrained manner, there would be an automatic improvement in all other aspects of life! What happened—because this theory became coupled with onrushing, unbridled capitalism—was that the ideal envisioned by Thomas Jefferson in the United States had been turned upside down. Instead of social progress being guided by such values as justice, freedom, and self-fulfillment for all people, rich or poor, these goals of vital interest in a democracy were subjugated to a burgeoning society dominated by supposedly more important *instrumental* or *material* values (i.e., useful or practical ones for advancing a capitalistic system).

So the fundamental question still today is, "which type of values will win out in the long run?" In North America, for example, it seems that a gradually prevailing concept of cultural relativism was increasingly discredited as the 1990s witnessed a sharp clash between (1) those who uphold so-called Western cultural values and (2) those who by their presence are dividing the West along a multitude of ethnic and racial lines. This multi–ethnicity is occasioning strong efforts to promote fundamental religions and sects—either those present historically or those recently imported legally or illegally–characterized typically by decisive right/wrong morality.

Postmodernism as an Influence

The orientation and review of selected world, European, North American, regional, and local developments occurring in the final quarter of the 20th century might seem a bit out of place to some who read this book. It could be asked whether this has a relationship to the value system in place in North America. My response to this question is a resounding "Yes." The affirmative answer is correct, also. if we listen to the voices of those in the minority within philosophy who are seeking to practice their profession, or promote their discipline as if it had some connection to the world as it exists. I am referring here, for example to a philosopher like Richard Rorty (1997).

He, as a so-called Neo-pragmatist, exhorts the presently "doomed Left" in North America to join the fray again. Their presumed shame should not be bolstered by a mistaken belief that only those who agree with the Marxist position that capitalism must be eradicated are "true Lefts." Rorty seems strongly concerned that philosophy once again become characterized as a "search for wisdom," a search that seeks conscientiously and capably to answer the myriad of questions looming before humankind all over the world.

While most philosophers have been "elsewhere engaged," what has been called postmodernism has become a substantive factor in intellectual circles. I must confess up front that I've been grumbling about—and seeking to grapple with—the term "postmodern" for years. Somehow it has now become as bad (i.e., misunderstood or garbled) as existentialism, pragmatism, idealism, etc.). I confess, also, that I have now acquired a small library on the topic. At any rate, when I first I read *Crossing the Postmodern Divide* by Albert Borgman (Chicago, 1992), I was so pleased to find something like this assessment of the situation. I say this because, time and again, I have encountered what I would characterize as gobbledygook describing what has been called "civilization's plight." By that I mean that what I encountered time and again was technical jargon, almost seemingly deliberately created obfuscation by people seemingly trying to "fool the public" on this topic. As I see it, if it's worth saying, it must be said carefully and understandably. Otherwise one can't help but think that the writer is a somewhat confused person.

At any rate, in my opinion this effort by Borgman is solid, down-to-earth, and comprehensible up to the final two pages. At that point he veers to Roman Catholicism as the answer to the plight of moderns. It is his right, of course, to state his personal opinion after describing the current situation so accurately. However, if he could have brought himself to it, or if he had thought it might be possible, I would have preferred it if he had spelled out several alternative, yet still other desirable directions for humankind to consider in the 21st century.

Is this modern epoch or era coming to an end? An epoch approaches closure when many of the fundamental convictions of its advocates are challenged by a substantive minority of the populace. It can be argued that indeed the world is moving into a new epoch as the proponents of postmodernism have been affirming over recent decades. Within such a milieu there are strong indications that all professions are going to have great difficulty crossing this so-called, postmodern gap (chasm, divide, whatever!). Scholars argue that many in democracies, under girded by the various rights being propounded (e.g., individual freedom, privacy), have come to believe that they require a supportive "liberal consensus" within their respective societies.

Post-modernists now form a substantive minority that supports a more humanistic, pragmatic, liberal consensus in society. Within such a milieu there are strong indications that present-day society is going to have difficulty crossing the "designated," postmodern divide. Traditionalists in democratically oriented political systems may not like everything they see in front of them today, but as they look elsewhere they flinch even more. After reviewing where society has been, and where it is now, two more questions need to be answered. Where is society heading? And. most importantly, where should it be heading?

Postmodernists subscribe largely to a humanistic, anthropocentric belief as opposed to a traditional theocentric position. They would subscribe, therefore, I believe, to what Berelson and Steiner in the mid-1960s postulated as a behavioral science image of man and woman. This view characterized human beings as a creatures continuously adapting reality to their own ends as the world "progressed" toward an indeterminate future (1964).

Thus, the authority of theological positions, dogmas, ideologies, and some "scientific infallibilism" is severely challenged. A moderate postmodernist—holding a position I feel able to subscribe to—that is I am able to bring "it all" into focus—would at least listen to what the "authority" had written or said before criticizing or rejecting it. A strong postmodernist goes his or her own way by early, almost automatic, rejection of tradition. Then this person presumably relies on a personal interpretation and subsequent diagnosis to muster the authority to challenge any or all icons or "lesser gods" extant in society.

If the above is reasonably accurate, it would seem that a postmodernist might well feel more comfortable by seeking to achieve personal goals through a modified or semi-postmodernistic position as opposed to the traditional stifling position of essentialistic theological realists or idealists. A more pragmatic "value-is-that-which-is proven-through-experience" orientation leaves the future an open-ended one for sure!

Whatever your personal orientation may be, you will be faced with decisions of varying complexity that must be made every day of your life.

How you make any such decisions will be based on a set of values "earned through existence not by inheritance"! Humans are "lurching ahead" with an ever-evolving value structure that they themselves are creating on a year-by-year basis. How frightening that is! How fortunate we are! (How I see it anyhow...)

PART III
Is Human Nature Predetermined?

A book describing how human physical activity in activities such as exercise and sport might be able to make a significant contribution toward eventual human survival on Earth might or might not be destined to make even the bottom rung of the bestseller list in a basically confused world. Yet, oddly enough, if such a book were well written and sufficiently informative, it *should actually* challenge the #1 spot. I write this because most of us know that the world is in "big trouble", *and yet practically no one is looking in this direction for any possible answers.*

The interesting thing is that people really should be looking in this direction for two pieces of advice. The first is that people in the "advanced" world *must* follow a wise pattern of "developmental physical activity" if they wish to live long, healthy, and satisfying lives. The second piece of advice is that people are neglecting the first piece of advice just mentioned and are *turning instead* to watching dubious types of involvement or "non-involvement" with innumerable competitive sports. Oh yes, they may occasionally get around to a bit of sporting exercise on a weekend, but to expect the majority to exercise *in the right way* regularly seems to out of the question or a "wishful dream" expressed to salve one's conscience. It is not that sport itself, or exercise, has unpleasant connotations–far from it. It's simply that sport is being "abused" or "maltreated" as people only watch it or use it incorrectly. As for as vigorous exercise is concerned, there are so many other "life activities" out there that the time never seems to be available if by chance the urge to participate is contemplated.

A logical progression on this subject would be to have an opening chapter that first asks the question: "What Is the Universe"? In other words, I should start from the very beginning! However, I didn't major in astronomy at my university. Even if I had done so, I probably would have had difficulty describing the universe to a generally educated reader. Frankly, I couldn't answer this question satisfactorily all by myself! So, I turned to Google on the Internet and simply typed "The Universe" in the line with the clicking cursor. As a result I discovered reams of information.

Now, if convenient, I urge you to do just that–right now! Unless I am mistaken, you will find two videos available to you in response. They are on either the first or second page that comes up. Click on the left one, the longer one that lasts about 10 minutes while playing good music. When I did this for the first time, I was completely overwhelmed by the unbelievable enormity of it all. All that I can say is: "Wow"! So, if you have a computer sleeping nearby, please do this. Then I truly think you will be more ready to start reading Part 1 below…

To continue: It would be a good bet that the large majority of people on Earth don't give much, if any, thought to the question "What Are Humans?" raised by the title of Part 1 above on the preceding page. We *are* humans: we *are* at the top of the food chain–and that's it! And yet *your* answer–and a *collective* answer to it–are absolutely vital and fundamental to our future on this very tiny planet in an unbelievably vast "multiverse". Living our lives from day to day we sometimes forget that the planet Earth originated more than 4 billion years ago—or maybe even earlier!.

Early man and woman, we are told, had their beginnings some one million years ago and have used crude tools for less than half that time. Three hundred thousand years have elapsed since the mutation of sub-man into man. We now know that many tribes roamed and then settled at various points in prehistoric Europe during a warming trend at the time of the Wurm Glaciation of the late Pleistocene Epoch from 35,000 to 25,000 years before the present.

The "Adventure of Civilization"

The adventure of civilization began to make some headway because of now-identifiable forms of early striving which embodied elements of great creativity (e.g., the invention of the wheel, the harnessing of fire). The subsequent development in technology, very slowly but steadily, offered humans some surplus of material goods over and above that needed for daily living. Nevertheless, the beginnings of the first civilizations as we know them are actually less than 10,000 years ago. (See, for example, *Bahn, 2000*.)

For example, the early harnessing of nature created the irrigation systems of Sumeria and Egypt, and these accomplishments led to the establishment of the first cities. Here material surpluses were collected, managed, and sometimes squandered; nevertheless, necessary early accounting methods were created that were subsequently expanded in a way that introduced writing to the human scene. As we now know, the development of this form of communication in time helped humans expand their self-consciousness and to evolve gradually and steadily in all aspects of culture. For better or worse, however, the end result of this social and material progress has created a mixed agenda characterized by good and evil down to the present. The prevailing religions are the product of the past 2,500 or so years. As types of political state go, democracy, is the youngest of infants, its official origins dating back only several centuries to the late 18th century. Is it any wonder that perfection appears to be a long way off?

On this subject Muller concluded that "the adventure of civilization is necessarily inclusive" (1952, p. 53). By that he meant that evil will probably always be with humankind to some degree, but it is civilization that sets the standards and then works to eradicate at least the worst forms of such evil. Racial prejudice, for example, must be overcome. For better or worse, there are now more than six billion people on earth, and that number appears to be growing faster than the national debt! These earth creatures are black-, yellow-, brown-, red-, and white-skinned, but basically we now know from genetic research that there is an "overwhelming oneness" in all humankind that we dare not forget (Huxley, 1967).

The Ways Humans Have Acquired Knowledge

Royce (1964) stated that there are notably four basic means whereby people sought to surmount the obstacles preventing them from acquiring fact, knowledge, and wisdomabout the universe, about Earth within it, and about people and other creatures residing on this planet:

(1) thinking, that has become known as
    rationalism
(2) intuiting or feeling, that is designated as
    intuitionism
(3) sensing, that means of knowing called
    empiricism
(4) believing, that tendency of humans to accept
    as truth that which is stated by a variety of
    presumably knowledgeable people—an
    approach known as authoritarianism

Four "Historical Revolutions" in the Development of the World's Communication Capability

As we move along with our consideration of the ongoing change that has taken place throughout history, the developments in communication are such that we humans can only marvel at the present status of opportunity for human growth that has been created. Isaac Asimov has delineated these stages as follows:

(1) the invention of speech,
(2) writing,
(3) mechanical reproduction of the printed word, and now
(4) to relay stations in space creating a blanketing communications network that is making possible a type of international personal relationship hitherto undreamed of by men and women (Asimov, 1970).

Humans we, who tend to think we are "the greatest," may be excused from wondering occasionally why the "Creator" took such a laborious route with many odd variations of flora and fauna to get to this point of "present greatness." For hundreds of thousands of years, the forebears of present-day humans chipped flints to their tools. However, as they used their brains and their hands, both an enormous biological advantage, it is now evident that in their primitive self-consciousness they were not living only for the moment like their contemporaries, the apes.

As various world evils are overcome or at least held in check, scientific and accompanying technological development will be called upon increasingly to meet the demands of the exploding population. Gainful work and a reasonable amount of leisure will be required for further development. Unfortunately, the necessary leisure required for the many aspects of a broad, societal culture to develop fully, as well as for an individual to grow and develop similarly within it, has come slowly. The average person in the world is far from acquiring full realization of such benefits. Why "the good life" for all has been seemingly so slow in arriving is not an easy question to answer. Of course, we might argue that times do change slowly, and that the possibility of increased leisure has really come quite rapidly once humans began to achieve some control of their environment.

Of course, there have been so many wars throughout history, and there has been very little if any let-up in this regard down to the present. Sadly, nothing is so devastating to a country's economy. Also, in retrospect, in the Middle Ages of the Western world the power of the Church had to be weakened to permit the separation of church and state. This development, coupled with the rising humanism of the Renaissance in the latter stages of that era, was basic to the rise of a middle class. Finally, the beginnings of the natural sciences had to be consolidated into real gains before advancing technology could lead the West into the Industrial Revolution (Toffler's "Second Wave").

Admittedly, permitting a conscious choice between alternatives goes so far as permitting the presence of "population pockets" where there is a demand to give creationism co-equal status with the teaching of a Darwinian long-range approach to human evolution in the schools. As humans we, who tend to think we are "the greatest," may be excused from wondering occasionally why the "Creator" took such a long and laborious route with so many odd variations of flora and fauna to get to this point of "present greatness." The power that these advantages provided humans was steadily combined with technological advancement, but somehow only offered minimal levels of freedom. As mentioned above, the early development of language as a means of communication was vitally important. This distanced sub–humans even more from the apes as cultural evolution became much faster than biological evolution. In a sense, culture brought with it "good news" and "bad news." The bad news was that humans are now to a large degree trapped in a world that they themselves created. Fixed habits and beliefs are strong inhibitors of change, growth, and what might be called progress.

The good news is that, very slowly, change did occur; growth did take place; and to most people such change and growth represented true progress. For example, prehistoric humans did interbreed, and in this way broadened their genetic base. In the final analysis this lends credence to the present-day argument introduced above that humans today—brown or yellow, black, and white—are indeed one race. This fact helps us to appreciate the development of worldwide cultural evolution. Unfortunately, however, progress has never been a straight-line affair. In the final analysis, this must be the answer for those of us who idealistically thought that the world would be in quite good shape by the year 2000! It may also provide some solace to those of us who wonder why education finds it so difficult to get sufficient funding; why professors in so many countries must often assume a "Rodney Dangerfield complex". Little wonder that physical activity education, including educational sport, despite consistently mounting evidence of the "worthwhileness" of developmental physical activity—so often finds itself in dire straits within the domain of education and in the eyes of the public.

World society is obviously in a precarious state. It is therefore important to view present social conditions globally. Throughout this volume I will be emphasizing that competitive sport has developed to a point where it has worldwide impact, and also human physical activity should be so organized and administered that it truly makes a contribution to what Glasser (1972) identified as "Civilized Identify Society"–a state in which the concerns of humans will again focus on such concepts as 'self-identity,' 'self-expression,' and 'cooperation.'

Postulating that humankind has gone through three stages of society already (i.e., primitive survival society, primitive identity society, and civilized survival society in which certain societies created conflict by taking essential resources from neighbors, Glasser theorized that the world should strive to move as rapidly as possible into a role-dominated society so that life as it is presently known can continue "wholesomely" on Earth.

Historical Images of Humans' Basic Nature

Any effort to delineate the present status of Western man and woman must include also some consideration of the postulations that have been offered concerning the basic nature of a human. In the mid-1950s, Van Cleve Morris presented a fivefold, chronological series of overlapping philosophical definitions including analyses as (1) a rational animal, (2) a spiritual being, (3) a receptacle of knowledge, (4) a mind that can be trained by usage and that functions within a body, and (5) a problem-solving organism (1956, pp. 22-22, 30-31). Within such a sequential pattern, the task of the physical activity educator/coach might be to help this problem-solving organism to move efficiently and with purpose in exercise, sport, and expressive movement. Of course, such experience would necessarily occur within the context of the individual's socialization in evolving world society.

A bit later, Berelson and Steiner (1964) traced six images of man and woman throughout history, but more from the standpoint of behavioral science than Morris' philosophically oriented definitions. These images were:

(1) The philosophical image (the equivalent of Morris' "rational animal"). In Classical Greece, ancient man and woman distinguished virtue through reason.

(2) The Christian image (Morris' "spiritual being") which contained the concept of "original sin" and the possibility of redemption through the transfiguring love of God for those who controlled their sinful impulses.

(3) The third image appearing in sequential order on the world scene during the Renaissance was the political image (a behavioral orientation in contrast to Morris' "receptacle of knowledge" a philosophical categorization), through which humans, through power and will, managed to take greater control of the social environment. In the process, sufficient energy was liberated to bring about numerous political changes, the end result being the creation of embryonic national ideals that co-existed with earlier religious ideals.

(4) The economic image of the human (contrasted this with Morris' "mind that can be trained by usage") emerged during the 18th and 19th centuries, one that provided an underlying rationale for economic development in keeping with the possession of property and material goods along with improved monetary standards.

(5) The psychoanalytic image emerged in the

early 20th century. Berelson and Steiner postulated the stage that was not included in Morris' classification. It introduced another form of love—that of self. Instinctual impulses were being delineated more carefully than ever before. The result was that people were led to believe that childhood experiences and other non-conscious controls often ruled people's actions because of the frequently incomplete gratification of basic human drives related to libido and sex.

(6) Finally, because of the rapid development of the behavioral sciences, they postulated the behavioral-science image of men and women (roughly the equivalent of Morris' "problem-solving organism," but with an added social dimension). This view of the human characterized him or her as a creature continuously adapting reality to his or her own ends. In this way the individual is seeking to make reality more pleasant and congenial and—to the greatest possible extent—his own or her own reality (Berelson & Steiner, 1964, pp. 662667).

Seven Rival Theories About Human Nature

Keeping Berelson and Steiner's six images of human nature listed above in mind, in trying to answer this question about human nature more precisely, I eventually decided to include further the insightful work of Leslie Stevenson. He suggested that there are at least seven rival theories that postulate an answer to this basic question about the basic or intrinsic nature of man (generically speaking) (1987). Each of these prognostications is saying in essence: This is "the hand that we've been dealt," and "this is how we can best react to it what it is telling us":

1. Plato: The Rule of the Wise
2. Christianity: God's Salvation
3. Marx: Communistic Revolution
4. Freud: Psychoanalysis

5. Sartre: Atheistic Existentialism
6. Skinner: The Conditioning of Behavior
7. Lorenz: Innate Aggression

As I continued, it seems that my purpose here will be best served as well by a brief consideration of each of the seven theories delineated by Stevenson about (1) the nature of the universe, (2) the nature of men, (3) a diagnosis of the situation humans face, and (4) a prescription of what each "prognosticator" thought should be done to bring about the best result.

Theory #1: Plato–The Rule of the Wise. Following the above sequence, Plato, for example, is arguing that that (1) this is my theory about the universe we live in (i.e., his theory of another world of "existing Forms"), (2) our nature as humans as being dualistic (i.e., mind and body), (3) the belief that these Forms are ideals about the parallel world, and (4) the prescription that the only way the world is going to "make it" is if the wisest of men rule it. (Note: I suppose in a way that's what we are doing in a democracy where we elect a person as head of state for a period of time…)

Theory #2: Christianity–God's Salvation. Moving ahead to theory #2, Stevenson stated next that Christianity also had a theory about (1) the nature of the universe, (2) what humans were like in this environment, (3) how God has explained what is wrong with man and women, and (4) what he/she needs to do about it to be saved. It does seem that there are so many differences and subdivisions by people subscribing to this theory that it is difficult to spell out the "essentials." God created the universe that is "up there" somewhere in space and in time. This universe is identified with God, a deity that is both transcendent and immanent.

The nature of man is explained as a creature made in the image of God and who is destined to have control of the rest of God's creation. However, in a seeming contradiction, he/she is also "continuous with it." True Christians believe there is life after death through a process of resurrection. A crucial point in Christianity's view of human nature is that the human is free and has the ability to love while finding true purpose (i.e., love of God).

Proceeding to the "diagnosis stage" of this theory, we find that the human has from the beginning misused his God-given right of free will by initially making the wrong choice. In this way he has sinned and the relationship with the Creator was upset. Hence, nothing he/she does will bring about "perfection" in life and living. The human alienated himself from God by assertion of the will.

What is the prescription then? Humans must look to God for ultimate salvation. The New Testament of *The Bible* helps humanity to find a way to eternal salvation by explaining that God sent his son, Jesus, to earth to restore the disturbed relationship that developed through suffering and atonement for the evil of man. Each person on earth must individually accept "God's redemption" provided to him/her by the life and resurrection of Jesus. In this way a way of life has been provided for the true believer.

Theory #3: Marx–Communist Revolution. It is interesting to note that Karl Marx was born a Jew in a German family that converted to Christianity. Eventually devoting himself to the philosophy of Hegel, Marx believed that humankind was destined to go through certain stages of development, each possessing a "character" of its own. This was in essence a pantheistic belief asserting that God was the whole of reality. However, when Hegel's followers split into two camps, Marx followed the thought of Feuerbach that led to the belief that religion was really identified with alienation from earthly affairs. Hence, he opted for a more radical position that it was up to humans to help move the development of humankind to a new stage of development that envisioned social progress yo be tied to material rather than spiritual progress. This resulted in the ongoing application of a materialistic interpretation of history that led to the rise of the interpretation of history as being too materialistic thereby leading to the idea that capitalism must be eliminated as the prevailing economic theory.

Marx claimed that his theory of the universe explained historical development scientifically; thus, he searched for universal laws underlying social development. An "Asiatic phase" gave way to an ancient era that eventually merged with a feudal period. Then a socialistic phase set in to be followed inevitably by a capitalistic one as worldwide commerce gradually developed. Ultimately, as we know, capitalism was to be forced to give way to communism. There were laws of history operating here, he claimed, arguing that this study of history was truly a science that could be tested by evidence. His theory appears to overemphasize the materialist conception of history asserting that material life's mode of production is what gives society its "character" socially, politically, and "spiritually.

Although capitalism has its problems, it is still in an extremely strong position in the world with some of the avowed communistic countries adopting many of its practices. However, this struggle is far from over as the gap between rich and poor accentuates with the middle class being squeezed increasingly between them in so-called developed countries. Thus, it could be argued that a type of socialism will be needed to satisfy "the multitudes in their search for a good life."

In the theory of man that is postulated with Marxism, the future is deterministic as man progresses through various stages of history being exhorted to help the process along. Some urge that the change be brought about precipitously, whereas others seem willing to let history evolve. The essentially social nature of the human is viewed as fundamental. We learn through our relationships with others. In addition, different from all other creatures, we have learned to produce a good deal of what is needed for our subsistence. Human development could be considered a social development brought about by men and women possessing a strong sense of social activism. The study of sociology is obviously extremely important.

Marx's diagnosis of the human's plight is that he/she (Western human actually) has become alienated within world society because of the gradual adoption of capitalism as the economic system to emulate. It is difficult to understand exactly how such alienation from one's self and Nature has occurred. However, we can assume that this alienation might be from what humanity has created, and this alienation is also from the basic nature of humans. It may be possible to get some help by looking to the main points of the *Communist Manifesto*. Difficulty arises, however, when we conjecture that Marx's concern would be nicely rectified by turning everything over to the State instead of leaving so much in the hands of private enterprise. However, we can understand that Marx was "loudly" decrying the abuses displayed in the early stage of capitalism when men served *only* as an economic end.

Moving from diagnosis to prescription with Theory #3 about human nature is a simple matter. An economic system where capitalism prevails is a bad development, and it must eliminated while something better is introduced. That "something" is to be "the Communist Revolution"! The debate really warms up at this point. Social democracy is too "gentle" and "long-winded" to bring about the necessary change; so, "bring on the Revolution"! The aftermath of this overthrow would be a social system in which humans would be "regenerated" and function in a society where ideally and eventually the State as supreme power would fade away. Considered in the light of day, we cannot but agree that the envisioned end is indeed glorious. However, considering the nature of the human, we must be suspicious of this demand to "throw out the baby with the bathwater and begin all over again." Nevertheless we know that a large segment of the world's population is living in societies that claims to have done just that…

Theory #4: Freud–Psychoanalysis. Sigmund Freud and his theory of psychoanalysis are important to us in this discussion because through his work he made such an enormous contribution to people's understanding of themselves as they live in an evolving world. Freud was a scientist who evidently didn't spend much time on metaphysical speculation about the nature of the universe, He was purported to be an atheist who viewed the world as a phenomenon in which such sub-phenomena are governed by what are called physics and chemistry. Humans evolved on this planet and are presumably subject to any laws that prevail.

The subject becomes much more complicated, however, when we shift our attention to humans. Stevenson decided to subsume Freud's ideas about humans under four categories: (1) application of the principle of determinism, (2) the postulation of unconscious mental states arising from the first category, (3) his theory of the instincts human instincts or "drives," and (4) his developmental theory of individual human character.

Determinism meant that every "mental event" was a result of something previous that occurred in the human mind. The second category delved into mental states by asserting that "the mind is not co-extensive with what is conscious or can become conscious." There are dynamic, unconscious aspects of the mind that can influence action. This does not mean, however, that a Platonic dualistic theory (mind/body) of the human is true; the principles of physiology still hold sway. He postulated, however, that the mind has three major structural systems: (the *id*, the *ego*, and the *super-ego*. The drives of the id need immediate satisfaction; the ego has to do with the human's relationship to the outside world and thereby has a direct influence on any possible anti-social drives, for example, of the id. The superego, as he postulates is that part of the ego that mediates between the outside world and the person's id. It seems confusing, but the task of the superego is to supervise the ego by projecting society's moral rules and norms to help the id "restrain itself" as the human faces society daily. Simple, n'est-ce pas?

As if this weren't enough for one man's theoretical contribution. Freud also opined about the great importance of instincts or "drives" as motivating forces within the human mind. The one that has received the most attention perhaps overemphasis, of course has to do with the human's sexual drive.

We can't leave our all-too-brief discussion of Freud's work without inclusion of Freud's developmental theory of the individual having to do with human character. He theorized about the respective influences of experience and heredity as the child and youth goes through the several stages of development on the way to maturity. It is obvious that Freud presented humanity with much to ponder over on the subject of human nature.

Moving to the "diagnosis stage" with this summary of Freud's contribution, it is immediately obvious that the well-adjusted person would exhibit a harmonious relationship among the various "parts" of the brain (as postulated by Freud) as the individual confronts "the outside world." A person can talk about it glibly using the terms supplied, we know that "making it all work" to the individual's and society's best interest is another matter. For example, there is the concept of "repression" that might be used as a defense mechanism when the person is under stress and can't seem to adjust to society's demands. However, as we mature, we must learn to cope with the conditions that confront us to "maintain control" within our familial and external environments. To what extent society "may have gone wrong" is another matter.

To undertake some "prescribing" after brief diagnosis, Freud would have us maintain a harmonious state between the several "parts" of the mind. In addition, there needs to be reasonable harmony between the person and the world. Freud did not get into the question of possible social reform, but devoted a large portion of his time and effort to the psychoanalysis of patients. Further discussion of this treatment would serve no purpose in this volume devoted to human values and disvalues related to sport and physical activity.

Theory #5: Sartre–Existentialism. Philosophers identified with what has been called existentialism are a "very mixed breed." However, there does appear to be consensus that this approach is concerned with the individual, the purpose of his/her life, and the amount of freedom granted to said person. Interestingly there are both Christian and atheistic existentialists!

Jean Paul Sartre's "brand" of existentialism denied the existence of a God, and he inquired as to what that "non-existence" meant for the individual human. Most importantly this theory of a God-free universe meant that there are no such things as "objective values" that control human life. Thus, if life has no purpose, Sartre described it as "absurd." For him this meant, therefore, that the individual is free to choose his/her life values.

How, therefore, do we describe the nature of this creature that has evolved and whom we call "man"? We are here. But there doesn't seem to be any reason for our presence. This means that, since we are sentient. if we are to have a purpose we had best get at its creation. Right now we really don't know what we ought to be! However, it does seem apparent that we have been "condemned to be free." So what are we going to do about it?

The result seems to be that the human been challenged with responsibility because of the freedom somehow granted to him or her. It's sort of a "don't just sit there; move it!" situation. Hence, what we do, or don't do, assumes great importance to ourselves–and to others who may be in our path as we wander through life.

The diagnosis of the plight that has befallen man is crucial. We can deceive ourselves and say we are not free, but that would be stupid. Sartre calls such deception "bad faith," but admits that many people end up trapped in their life situations in this way.

Unfortunately, however, the rejection of the bad-faith approach does not offer the human a clear and definitive assessment of the self. Defining the self is truly elusive, because, as Stevenson (p. 97) asserts: "human reality is not *necessarily* what it is, but must be *able* to be what it is not." This seems to boil down to a case of "striving mightily" to be truly free and in the process to avoid "bad faith."

Okay… Where does this leave us when we come to the question of prescription for the individual subscribing to the existentialistic stance in life? The situation is that there are no basic values so far as we can see. So we have to figure what life amounts to all by ourselves. As an individual, therefore, I should try to avoid "bad faith" and do my level best to be "authentic" in whatever I choose to do with my life. This is the challenge handed over to us if we accept this philosophical stance. So be it!

Theory #6: Skinner–The Conditioning of Behavior. To this point the efforts included have been those of men approaching the question of human nature philosophically to a large degree. The next one included here takes a somewhat more scientific tack into what has become the discipline of psychology. Here we will condense very briefly the efforts of B. F. Skinner, an experimental psychologist, studies that led him to make generalizations about human nature from the area known as "the behaviorist tradition."

Skinner was preceded in his endeavors by J. B. Watson and others who sought to carry out their research empirically as "the study of consciousness." However, Skinner in a 1913 paper stated that they\se scholars had reached the point where they could not agree on methodology in their research. Hence, he argued that it was time to "go outwards" and study human *behavior*. It could be observed and analyzed better than the assessment of previous introspective analyses. In addition, the importance of environment in human development, as over against heredity, was singled out by Skinner. This question is still open, however, in the 21ˢᵗ century.

With regard to *the theory of* the universe underlying Skinner/s approach, his endeavor was simply an affirmation of thought stating that scientific method must be used to determine what nature, including human nature is all about. The search must be for uniformities and general laws that apply under all circumstances. In this way theory grows and expands as the human seeks to control the environment and thereby thrive on into the indeterminate future. At present people make value judgments and then seek to induce others to accept their stated position on "this and that" about the world. If some practice works efficiently. And effectively (beneficently) in society, that means it should be evaluated as "good." To summarize, Skinner as a scientist was searching for uniformities among phenomena looking to understanding, relating, and ultimately controlling the world.

Insofar as Skinner's study of human nature went, he viewed the individual as a whole–not as some "metaphysically dualistic creature" that is literally "unexplainable". Keeping genetic factors in mind, he looked for environmental causation of human behavior. He believed (1) that there were scientific laws to be determined that governed human behavior, and (2) that these laws explain the relationship between these environmental factors and subsequent human behavior. In assessing these statements, we are somehow left, however, with the possibility that analysis of behavior doesn't "explain it all"–that there may also be "innate factors" that come into play as well.

Reflecting on a *diagnosis* of Skinner's theory, we are confronted with the clash between his thought and that of Sartre. Skinner believes in the determinism "of it al," and Sartre tell us that we are "condemned to be free"! Are humans "free agents" or not? What a difficult question to answer! And yet we might as well "throw in the towel" if we concur with Skinner in this regard. On the other hand, however, the "loneliness" of the person in the world postulated by Sartre is "scary" as well. Whether an intermediate position is possible appears to be the question. If there was a "social cause" for my "dubious action," why can't I be held at least partially responsible by society?

Now let us consider the *prescription* stage in regard to Skinner's deterministic position at hand. The human is faced with a world that "determines" where he/she is heading. Much of this looks very worrisome indeed. Do we "give in to it," or do we work mightily to create a situation where we find longevity and "life satisfaction" as the world evolves? Skinner would have us improve the present situation by conditioning people's behavior in a variety of ways (i.e., inducements, "positive" propaganda). This all sounds most encouraging. However, there is just "one hitch"! Someone, or some group of people, would have to "call the shot," so to speak. This is indeed a tricky situation in which to be placed. I, as author, find myself of two mind as to my decision. Finally, I must opt for "the dignity of freedom to choose myself"!

Theory #7: Lorenz–Innate Aggression. Finally in this "you pay your money; you take your choice approach" I am offering here, we come to the work of Konrad Lorenz, a man who called himself an ethologist and argued that the happenings of early childhood are basic to a person's subsequent philosophical and later scientific development. This attempt to study the character of animals scientifically by describing what happens when the environmental situation of creatures changes or is altered.

The assumption was that the instinctual behavior patterns of a particular species occurred as a result of the individual's genes evolving down through the ages. Hence it is easy to understand why Darwin's *Origin of Species* (1859) caused such a furor when the human's evolution through so-called natural selection was propounded. I won't attempt to repeat the four empirical propositions tested by this assertion. Suffice it to say that "the world" has not been the same since this contradiction of Christian doctrine.

As the work of Lorenz proceeded, he concentrated on the aggressive behavior of humans and what this meant for "the human condition." Hence as this biological scientist considered the nature of the universe, he found that creatures of this Earth had developed hereditary movements that were instinctive and innate even though many of these human creatures' drives gave the appearance of spontaneity. The four most important drives of feeding, reproduction, flight, and aggression combined to provide a sort of unity to human nature.

Here Lorenz's special study of human aggression is being considered—a major instinctive drive. He examined how various species had learned to "protect their territory" in order to survive down through the ages. The "necessary" aggression had its bad points and its good points, as Lorenz saw it, but overall under "controlled circumstances" such aggression may be desirable when not overly destructive.

Moving along to Lorenz's theory of human nature, it is obvious that it correlates strongly to behavior patterns exhibited by other animals. Nature's causal laws work on us too, and we deny this similarity to out individual and collective peril. This doesn't mean, however, that some people have not developed a high degree of personal control in regard to their aggressive nature. A highly interesting theory emerges from his deliberations and studies, however. Somehow we appear to have developed an almost innate drive leading to aggression toward our own species—perhaps even more so than is the case with many other animals! This came about possibly when other tribes threatened a specific tribe, and over the millennia the "warrior instinct" emerged as basic to survival. Certain types of "communal defense" may have preordained people to aggression for survival purposes.

The diagnosis of this development postulated by Lorenz may mean that literally weak human insofar as possessing deadly appendages were concerned had no need to worry especially about "human internecine warfare" before the "age of deadly weapons" appeared to present humankind with the possibility of complete annihilation and self-destruction. Hence, we seem to have ended up with a situation where one society can cause mass destruction of another—something completely out of the question and impossible for other species. (This may be a good reason for humans to follow the advice of Dr. Hawking that earthlings shouldn't ne in too big a hurry to relate to species on other planets!)

Proceeding to what might be a possible prescription for the human being who conceivably might have acquired through the passage of eons an innate aggressiveness toward his *"foreign"* neighbor in a circumscribed world where "neighbors" are within easy striking distance, what can be recommended? Might it be possible somehow to eliminate this frightening aggression? We can't build impregnable walls, nor can we drugs that will pacify us. If one culture were to try to "breed aggression out" of its population, who's to say that other groupings would reciprocate? It seems that only more self–knowledge resulting from research might help people understand their feelings and motivations better. In this way we might promote significant good will leading to international peace.

Interestingly, and hopefully, there were groups of British and American scientists, lead by M. F. Ashley Montagu and others who argued conversely against the man-is-bad view of humankind. They argue that the question is still debatable, far from having been decided convincingly that the future looks bleak for the human species. Undoubtedly the twentieth century has been a bleak one, and the beginning of the twenty-first one hasn't seen many positive signs yet of a new, more peaceful age. However, we must proceed on the basis that "there is hope yet" for a more peaceful world in the future.

Two Basic Historical Questions

To this point we know that we are organisms, living creatures, who have reached a stage of development where we "know that something has happened, is continuing to happen, and will evidently continue to happen." However, underlying my entire analysis I am searching for the answers to *two historical questions*: First, did humans in earlier times, equipped with their coalescing genes and evolving **memes,** enjoy to any significant degree what discerning people today might define as "quality living?"

(Note: Memes are sets of "cultural instructions" passed on from one generation to the next; see below, also.)

Second, did earlier humans have an opportunity for freely chosen, beneficial physical activity in sport, exercise, play, and dance of sufficient quality and quantity to contribute to the quality of life (as viewed possible by selected sport philosophers today)?

(Note: Of course, the phrasing of these questions—whether humans in earlier societies enjoyed quality living, including fine types of developmental physical activity—is no doubt presumptuous. It reminds one of the comedian whose stock question in response to his foil who challenged the truth of the zany experiences his friend typically reported: "Vas you dere, Sharlie?")

What makes a question about the quality of life in earlier times doubly difficult, of course, is whether present-day humans can be both judge and jury in such a debate. On what basis can we decide, for example, whether any social progress has indeed been made such that would permit resolution of such a concept as "quality living" including a modicum of "ideal sport competition" or "purposeful physical activity and related health education."?

There has been progression, of course, but how can we assume that change is indeed progress? It may be acceptable as a human criterion of progress to say that we are coming closer to approximating the good and the solid accomplishments that we think humans should have achieved both including what might be termed "the finest type" of sport competition.

The Difficulty of Defining Progress

Despite what has just been stated above the "forward leaps" that have been made in the area of communication, any study of history inevitably forces a person to conjecture about human progress. I first became truly interested in the concept of progress when I encountered the work of the world-famous paleontologist, George Gaylord Simpson (1949, pp. 240-262). After 25 years of research, he offered his assessment of the question whether evolution represented progress. His study convinced him that it was necessary to reject "the over-simple and metaphysical concept of a pervasive perfection principle." That there had been progression he would not deny, but he inquired whether this really was progress. The difficulty comes, he argued, when we assume that change is progress; we must ask ourselves if we can recommend a criterion by which progress may be judged.

We are warned that it may be shortsighted for us to be our own "judge and jury" in this connection. It may well be an acceptable human criterion of progress to say that we are coming closer to approximating what we think we ought to be and to achieving what we hold to be good. It is not wise, according to Simpson, however, to automatically assume that this is "the only criterion of progress and that it has a general validity in evolution." Thus, throughout the history of life there have been examples of progress and examples of retrogression, and progress is "certainly not a basic property of life common to all its manifestations." If it is a materialistic world, as Simpson would have us believe, a particular species can progress and regress. There is "a tendency for life to expand, to fill in all the space in the livable environments," but such expansion has not necessarily been constant, although it is true that human beings are now "the most rapidly growing organism in the world."

It is true also that we have made progress in adaptability and have developed our "ability to cope with a greater variety of environments." This is also progress considered from the human vantage point. The various evolutionary phenomena among the many species, however, do not show "a vital principle common to all forms of life," and "they are certainly inconsistent with the existence of a supernal perfecting principle." Thus, Simpson concludes, human progress is actually relative and not general, and "does not warrant choice of the line of man's ancestry as the central line of evolution as a whole." Yet it is safe to say that "man is among the highest products of evolution… and that man is, on the whole but not in every single respect, the pinnacle so far of evolutionary progress" on this Earth.

With the realization that evolution (of human and other organisms) is going on and will probably continue for millions of years, we can realize how futile it is to attempt to predict any outcome for the ceaseless change so evident in life and its environment. We can say that we must be extremely careful about the possible extinction of our species on Earth, because it is highly improbable, though not absolutely impossible, that our development would be repeated. Some other mammal might develop in a similar way, but this will not happen so long as we have control of our environment and do not encourage such development. Our task is to attempt to modify and perhaps to control the direction of our own evolution according to our highest goals. It may be possible through the agency of education, and the development of a moral sense throughout the world, to ensure the future of our species; one way to accomplish this would be to place a much greater emphasis on the social sciences and humanities while working for an ethically sound world-state at the same time.

The "Tragic Sense of Life" (Muller)

One realizes immediately, also, that any assessment of the quality of life in prerecorded history, including the possible role of sport in that experience, must be a dubious evaluation at best. However, I was intrigued by the work of Herbert Muller who has written so insightfully about the struggle for freedom in human history. I was impressed, also, by his belief that recorded history has displayed a "tragic sense" of life. Whereas the philosopher Hobbes (1588-1679) stated in his *De Homine* that very early humans existed in an anarchically individualistic state of nature in which life was "solitary, poor, nasty, brutish, and short," Muller (1961) argued in rebuttal that it "might have been poor and short enough, but that it was never solitary or simply brutish" (p. 6).

Accordingly, Muller's approach to history is "in the spirit of the great tragic poets, a spirit of reverence and or irony, and is based on the assumption that the tragic sense of life is not only the profoundest but the most pertinent for an understanding of both past and present" (1952, p. vii). The rationalization for his "tragic" view is simply that the drama of human history has truly been characterized by high tragedy in the Aristotelian sense. As he states, "All the mighty civilizations of the past have fallen, because of tragic flaws; as we are enthralled by any Golden Age we must always add that it did not last, it did not do" (p. vii).

This made me wonder whether the 20th century of the modern era might turn out to be the Golden Age of the United States. This may be true because so many misgivings are developing about former blind optimism concerning history's malleability and compatibility in keeping with American ideals. As Heilbroner (1960) explained in his 'future as history' concept, America's still-prevalent belief in a personal "deity of history" may be short-lived in the 21st century. Arguing that technological, political, and economic forces are "bringing about a closing of our historic future," he emphasized the need to search for a greatly improved "common denominator of values" (p. 178).

However, all of this could be an oversimplification, because even the concept of 'civilization' is literally a relative newcomer on the world scene. Recall that Arnold Toynbee (1947) came to a quite simple conclusion about human development is his monumental *A study of history*—that humankind must return to the one true God from whom it has gradually but steadily fallen away. An outdated concept, you might say, but there is a faint possibility that Toynbee may turn out to be right. However, we on this Earth dare not put all of our eggs in that one basket. We had best try to use our heads as intelligently and wisely as possible as we get on with striving to make the world as effective and efficient—and as replete with good, as opposed to evil, as we possibly can.

Here we might well be guided by the pact that Goethe's *Faust* made with the Devil. In this literary masterpiece from the pen of the German literary figure, Johann Wolfgang von Goethe (1748-1832), we recall the essence of the agreement struck by Faust with the then-presumed actual purveyor of the world's evil. If ever the time were to come when Faust was tempted to feel completely fulfilled and not bored by the power, wealth, and honor that the horned one had bestowed upon him, then the Devil would have won, and accordingly would have the right to take him away to a much warmer climate. Eventually, as the reader may recall, by conforming to the terms of the agreement, Faust is saved by the ministrations of the author. Yet, we at present can never forget for a moment that previous human civilizations were not miraculously saved! Literally, not one has made it! Thus, "Man errs, but strive he must," admonished Goethe, and we as world citizens today dare not forget that dictum.

Postscript

With some trepidation I decided to add a short postscript to Part III in I have discussed human nature. After seven years of working full time in physical education and athletics beginning in 1941, I was still taking graduate courses here and there as I worked my way along laboriously looking to the doctoral degree. In a 1947-48 graduate course at Columbia Teachers College, at the behest of Dr. Josphine Rathbone, my instructor, I published my first article in a professional journal. Interestingly, it was titled "Implications of the study of body types for physical education" (*JOPERD, 15, 3:240-42, 254.*).

I was fascinated with the work of Dr. William H. Sheldon and colleagues that was explained in their publication titled *The Varieties of Human Physique* (1940). Sheldon was interested in the relationships between physique, psychology and delinquency. The word "somatotype" was invented to describe a human body type that had three components that could be assessed on 7-point scales (i.e., "endomorphy", "mesomorphy", and" ectomorphy". The somatotype assigned after examination was presumably unchangeable with the components being derived from original "embryonic layers". In the human embryo there are three layers of cells known as the endoderm, the mesoderm, and the ectoderm

Sheldon created quite a stir with this assessment of the human body–a so-called "constitutional approach" that postulated differing levels of "involvement" of each of the three components in a human being. For example, an individual heavy in the mesomorphic component, and lower in the other two might rate a 2-7-2 analysis. A problem arose when he argued the permanence of such a rating once determined. This position was challenged seriously. Subsequently, when he and S.S. Stevens produced *The Varieties of Temperament* that sought to link or correlate the three-pronged, individual analysis of somatype with this or that specific human temperament or nature, the scientific world quickly speedily reacted negatively. So it looks as if we are on "shaky ground" if we should attempt to make direct assumptions about human *nature* (including behavior) from *bodily somatotype*…

PART IV
The Status of Physical Activity Education and Sport

Introduction

Physical activity education, *including* what is here called sport, is a field that in the 21st century is facing one more crossroad in its torturous historical development. As it happened, after approximately 200 years, during which time people were involved in subsistence physical activity and indigenous physical recreation and games, some nineteenth-century European leaders in organized physical activity brought their varying ideas about physical training and gymnastics to the "New World."

Those directing the effort after the American Civil War adopted the name "physical education" with a new national association founded in the 1880s. What then gradually developed on this soil has been termed a unique "American system" of physical education. Over the decades of the 20th century, this "American program" has included the following to greater or lesser extent: (1) elements of health and safety education, (2) physical education, (3) physical recreation, (4) sport, and (5) dance

As it developed, since the founding of the Association for the Advancement of Physical Education in 1985 (AAHPERD today), the field of physical activity education (including sport) has had many obstacles to overcome. *Sadly, yet interestingly, despite the enormous importance of what the field has to offer humankind, American society faces a predicament that is not recognized by the large majority of the population. People just don't seem to fully comprehend the seriousness of the situation!*

The fact is that the field of physical activity education (and related school health & safety education) is not receiving the support and attention it needs (and warrants!) to serve children, youth, and young adults adequately–and certainly not fully. It appears that the public doesn't recognize this situation or, to the extent that it does, does not believe it is worth the attention and expense of doing anything significant to rectify the problem.

A major aspect of the predicament relates to the evolving role of sport in society. Sport has become a social institution that is accepted in its many forms without being required to prove itself worthwhile and beneficial. Somehow sport is developing "relentlessly" in ways that should cause the discerning onlooker to question whether it is producing more "good" than "bad" in the culture. Sport has become an ever-present factor in the daily lives of the developed world. However it is functioning with no underlying theory that is being even semi-scientifically affirmed as it evolves. People think, generally speaking, that sport involvement is good for children, youth, and young adults. The prevailing credo is: "The more involvement there is in sport, the better off people *and* society will be." However, I believe this rosy picture painted is becoming dimmer with each passing day…

Both of these predicaments should be resolved as soon as it is humanly possible. However, the "powers that be" will have to be convinced about the necessity for such action before we can expect change to occur. The situation is complex and seemingly difficult to explain because it is compounded by its relationship with democracy, nationalism, and capitalism. Despite the prediction that youth of the oncoming generation will die at an earlier age than their parents, or the assertion that overly organized competitive sport appears may be doing more harm than good in a variety of ways, the large majority of the population is not ready to demand: (1) that in a variety of ways sanity should be restored to competitive sport because it has "lost its way," and (2) that a required, daily, physical activity education (and related health education program) is needed throughout the educational system at all levels. (In addition to the gymnasium-oriented program, a supplementary, intramural competitive–sport program is needed for both "normal" and "special-needs" children and youth.

To discuss further such a glaring omission in our educational system, I ask why we then turn around and devote an enormous amount of time, effort, and money to promote "varsity sport for the few"? I can see no justifiable reason to continue with the present approach unless the urgent needs of the mass of students are first met. If we are honest and fair, this situation must change at the first possible moment. The only conclusion I can come to is the following: *"Sport does not equate with [a fine program of] physical activity education and related health education. A varsity team program for accelerated children and youth should be made available only after the physical activity education needs of the large majority of youth have been met!*

As you catch your breath, while contemplating the uproar that the instigation of such a proposal would produce, I can appreciate that this may seem to be a ridiculous assertion on a continent where competitive sport has become such a powerful social institution. Nevertheless, I simply ask this question: "In what other aspect of the entire educational program do we take care of the needs and wishes of a tiny minority of the school population to the detriment of the large majority of the students?

As it developed historically, this unique situation occurs only in North America! Nowhere else in the world do we find that a competitive athletics program has become an institution for the "physically gifted" within the schools at the middle-school, secondary, and tertiary educational levels. Competitive sport, although popular around the world, has never been accepted as part of the educational program such as academic subjects are.

Of course, you may reply: "Competitive sport hasn't been accepted as part of the official *educational* program here either!" This is true, but somehow it has assumed a place of importance despite the fact that its importance of its contribution cannot be verified. It is a social institution without an accompanying theory that is supported by evidence. In addition, as a matter of fact, there is now solid evident that such desirable traits a honesty, fair play, truth, and sportsmanship decline the longer that athlete continues with sport competition! (This to me was a "clincher"...)

"A disastrous mistake"? "Crisis, what crisis?" you may ask. My response is: "It's getting closer, and it's really going to really bite you, if you don't look out!" Face it! Anyway one wants to look at it, the handwriting is on the wall! North American children and youth are simply not getting regular, quality physical activity education programs throughout their entire educational experience. The result is going to be that they will "pay for it" sooner *and* later. And we, members of the general public, are really going to pay for it later in horrendous health costs and in several other vital ways.

And sadly, we will have no one else to blame but ourselves because we are being warned, and we had been forewarned down through the years. In September, 2004, The Centers for Disease Control and Prevention of the United States released a report titled "Participation in High School Physical Education–United States, 1991-2003" (*MMWR Weekly*, Sept, 17, 2004 / 53(36), 844-847). In essence it states the evolving situation is not good, and that "If the national health objectives are to be achieved, coordinated efforts involving schools, communities, and policy makers are needed to provide daily, quality PE for all youth" (p. 1).

Next, on May 10, 2006, a significant article written by Eleanor Randolph was published in *The New York Times* titled "The Big, Fat American Kid Crisis . . .And 10 Things We Can Do About It". In this highly significant article, Ms. Randolph pointed out clearly and starkly that "Over the last 30 years. *obesity rates* have doubled among pre-schoolers and tripled for those age 6 to 11." After stating "Childhood obesity has become a medical crisis," she explains further that "The *National Institutes of Health* estimates that *Americans will take five years off our average lifespan* in a few years if we don't curb obesity, especially among the young." Still further, "The Centers for Disease Control and Prevention has estimated that this obesity epidemic is already costing our health care system about $79 billion a year."

Further, the June 2009 issue of the *Research Digest* of the President's Council on Physical Fitness and Sports (Series 10, No. 2) included a report titled " School Physical Education as a Viable Change Agent to Increase School Physical Activity. The summary statement in the article, written by Professors V. Gregory Payne, San Jose State University, CA and James R. Morrow, Jr. University of North Texas, Denton, stressed that:

> School physical education has been promoted by numerous expert sources as one of the most promising interventions in our nation's battle against physical inactivity, obesity, and morbidities. However, much room remains for improvement. Changes to the curriculum with the adoption of standards and enforcement of state policies can make school physical education one of the most powerful change agents for the serious health concerns facing our country.

Still further, on July 2, 2009, the Trust for America's Health (TFAH) and the Robert Wood Johnson Foundation (RWJF) followed up with "F as in Fat 2009 (How Obesity Policies are Failing in America"). Their findings are even more stark and foreboding: "Adult obesity rates increased in 23 states and did not decrease in a single state in the past year." Calling for a National Strategy to Combat Obesity that urges the defining of "roles and responsibilities for federal, state, and local governments" as well as "promoting collaboration among businesses, communities, schools, and families," A number of basic policies are recommended. Number #3 in this list states: "Increase the frequency, intensity, and duration of physical activity at schools."

Finally. a report from the National Association for Sport and Physical Education (NASPE) and the American Heart Association does show a slight improvement in the state of "PE" since the last such "Shape of the Nation" survey four years ago. There is some good news because the percentage of states requiring physical education has increased at the elementary, junior-high and high-school levels. However, the Report also states that most states don't (1) specify how much time should be allotted to such instruction and (2)–most unfortunately–about half of the states permit a variety of substitutions, exemptions, and waivers in connection with the requirement!

Nevertheless, this latest report (*2010 Shape of the Nation Report*) repeats the strong message that there is an urgent need to improve the overall quality of physical activity education programs including all aspects of "the health, academic performance, and well-being of all children and adolescents." (To download the complete report visit: www.naspeinfo.org/shapeofthenation.)

> N.B.: The "idea of parents setting an example for youth" becomes tricky when–as these words are being entered–the latest report from Statistics Canada indicated that only one in seven adults in Canada gets sufficient exercise!

Canadian Fitness Level. The situation in Canada is becoming drastic as well according to a report issued by Statistics Canada on January 15, 2010. (Steve Miller/Associated Press):

> "The results demonstrate a significant deterioration since 1981, regardless of sex or age. In particular, muscular strength and flexibility have decreased, and all measures of adiposity [fat] have increased," the authors of the report on children's fitness levels concluded.

Evidently, only one in right Canadian kids get enough exercise, a report by André Picard, Public Health Reporter, says in the *Globe and Mail* on Apr. 27, 2010.

See:
http://www.theglobeandmail.com/life/health/only-1-in-8-canadian-kids-get-enough-exercise-report-says/article1547931/

It is obvious that the die has been cast. We in the field of physical activity education must step up to the plate more than we have ever done so in the past. We can no longer permit colleagues in other fields and disciplines to downgrade the value of our potential contribution to the lives of children, youth, and young adults. The solution for us is to relate to all those groups mentioned above to help us make our case in both the public sector and in academe.

In doing so, we should state loudly and clearly: "We undertake physical activity regularly ourselves; we teach it to others; we teach other how to teach it; we research all aspects physical activity; and we administer programs of physical activity at all educational levels." (At the university level, if we don't think physical activity education sounds sufficiently "academic," we can say that our concern is with "developmental physical activity in exercise, sport, and related expressive activity".) Finally, it should be obvious that a full understanding of such involvement in human movement depends on knowledge emanating from the physical sciences, the social sciences, and the humanities.

A Terrible Predicament

As mentioned above briefly, America–the whole North American continent probably–got itself into such a predicament quite naturally as the population increased and urban centers developed. Historically, as the American Association for the Advancement of Physical Education (1885) "subdivided" and eventually became AAHPERD (and even spawned ICHPER-SD internationally), most of those "sub-divided" folks (e.g., health education, recreation) blithely went their own way as PE despite the valiant efforts of many "stumbled along" as the afterthought in the educational system. In Canada the earlier professional association became CAHPERD eventually, also, *until* it recently became Physical & Health Education Canada (PHE Canada)–a good move, I say.

This "name business" (i.e. deciding on the right name and sticking with it!) has been "driving me crazy and our field crazy" since I first became involved in the early 1940s. More recently I have been recommending the name *"physical activity education including educational sport"* for the "profession" and *"developmental physical activity"* as a name for any university unit. The recent trend, however, has been in the direction of adopting "kinesiology" as a disciplinary title. (This term may only confuse the public further, but it will probably help at the university level when professors apply fr research grants!)

Thinking historically and more broadly, however, physical education as a name for the field has indeed turned out to be a "bloody misnomer"! It was so, because–soon after the term "physical education" was adopted–psychological research in the early 20th century demonstrated that we are indeed *unified* organisms, the field of general education was thereby told that *henceforth* there couldn't be three separate types of education (i.e., physical, mental, and spiritual)!

In addition, because of the historical mind-body dichotomy dating back to the ancient Greek, Plato, and the "power of the church" subsequently, our field of physical education was "assigned" lower status automatically with this tri-partite educational philosophy (e.g., witness the place of "the body" in the well-known YMCA triangle!).

Further, in North America, Britain's "sporting tradition" began to develop in the mid-1800s. It had to compete with the foreign systems of gymnastics and exercise brought over from Europe. This might have worked out just fine, *if such activity had been introduced wholeheartedly within the educational curriculum on a regular basis.* However, it was deemed "extra-curricular" by educational essentialists–and resultantly has suffered from "second-class status" ever since.

There Is No Profession of Physical Education!. Shifting back to what *did* happen to what was called *physical* education within education, I recommend that now–after proclaiming it loudly for 100 years–the field should stop talking about the *profession* of physical education. We must do this because *we* ("PAE") are *not* a profession! We as individuals *are* professional *educators* responsible for physical activity education within the school curriculum.

In addition, related health and safety education is involved, although we are *not* typically fully qualified school health educators. School health education is far too important to be allotted as a second-hand responsibility of the physical activity educator. We are further typically not *professional* coaches, although based on background and training in selected sports, we carry out this function at the various educational levels. *Certainly we in physical activity education are not considered a separate profession by the public!*

Further, our frequent placement within departments, schools, or faculties of education at the university level (i.e., not as separate units in either the USA or Canada, for example) has somehow come to mean that our status is "automatically the 'lowest of the low' in the 'academic firmament'." I won't go into the history of this declaration at this point right now. That is just "the way it is out there"!

(Note: Many of physical education's professional programs in the United States are under the aegis of schools of education except where they managed to "escape" at some point historically. Even then, aspiring physical educators must have certain course experiences within the education unit on a campus to qualify for teacher status at the state level. The arrangement differs In Canada from province to province. In Ontario, for example, a separate degree is awarded (B.Ed.) after the baccalaureate degree in the field of physical education or kinesiology.

To broaden the outlook: Any idea of being a profession in society at large, in addition to being a professional educator responsible for physical activity education, "got away" from the field of physical education years ago and probably can never be retrieved. There are so many different professions or occupations "out there" whose practitioners promote this or that type of physical activity that to organize them "under one roof and one title" seem inconceivable. It might be worth a try, but it is "so late in the game." Thus, here we are today, as Jimmy Durante (the late comedian) was wont to say– *because the right kind of physical activity has proven to be such a good thing*– "Everybody wants to get in on the act!" And that's exactly what has been happening…

Just imagine it. Even many medics in the mid-20th century were almost "our enemies"; now they are proclaiming the benefits of physical activity daily as the beneficial results of this or that research project are reported. Of course, they should be doing just that! Why? Because we now know that "womb to tomb", developmental physical activity will not only help a person live life more fully, it will also help him or her to live longer! And yet, *somehow* (!) here we as physical activity educators are–at the beginning of the 21st century–with *inadequate* programs of physical and health education at all educational levels!

In addition, at the same time, *somehow* (!) commercialized, overemphasized, competitive sport is running rampant both within many high schools, colleges, and universities as well as "out there" in the public sector (including the Olympics). This is actually hurting our field of physical activity education and related health education because of the misplaced expenditure of energy and the accompanying "misdirected" use of available funding in communities across the North American continent. The situation has developed (retrogressed?) to the point where the "wrong" types of sporting experiences are promoted and actually "glorified"! A case can be made to the effect that because of such misplaced emphasis that competitive sport is probably doing more harm than good in world culture.

How Did This Come About Historically?

I found myself hard pressed to explain fully and correctly how this "tale of woe" came to be historically. Then I recalled VanderZwaag's analysis about what occurred during the period from 1880-1920 in the United States (1975). He had explained: "the nineteenth century was characterized by sectional interests and struggles among systems in physical education. This would not seem to be true today. What was the turning point?" VanderZwaag found the answer in "the steadily increasing interest in sports among the American people. The popularity of athletic contests was evident long before 1880. However, the earliest interest was developed through athletic clubs and intercollegiate athletics. The mass of the people did not receive the educational benefits to be derived from such activity."

As it turned out, the English sporting pattern won out over the several foreign systems of physical education. As VanderZwaag explained further that by 1920, it was evident that the United States had evolved a program of physical education that was characterized by informality and emphasis upon national sports. Such a program was thought to be entirely natural in view of our changing educational and political philosophies. Educationally, there was a growing recognition that a sound program of education should be based upon the needs of the child. This was also being recognized in the field of physical education that rapidly came to a system of physical education for the public schools that was based upon the play activities of childhood.

Why did this acceptance of "play and sport" as "physical education" materialize, you may ask? Seeking to answer this question more fully, I remembered that many years ago, when I was thesis adviser to the late Phyllis J. Hill at the University of Illinois, UIUC, Dr. Hill had provided an explanation in her investigation completed in 1965 (*A Cultural History of Sport in Illinois, 1673-1820*). In her concluding statement, she wrote: "I am forced to the position that American cultural practices, including sport, have been forged by environmental forces, rather than by Anglo-Saxon tradition". This conclusion has merit still today because as she explained further, "work ethics and sport ethics are so close as to be virtually indistinguishable."

I sought to comprehend what this means for us today in the field of physical (activity) education and (educational) sport. Hill had concluded: "if all human behavior is, indeed, a total and patterned response, *the understanding of sport can be furthered only when it is studied in reference to other human variables within the culture*" [the emphasis is by EFZ]. What can I conclude? I can only affirm that our goal was sound. However, other societal influences were brought to bear on the ideal thereby perverting it. Our task in physical activity education and educational/recreational sport is to help *all* people of all ages and conditions understand how important it is for them to be involved in a type of developmental physical activity that will enable them to *live life more fully* based on their choice of "life values." If they choose correctly, and we in the field help them to acquire the needed knowledge and skills to live life more fully, the evidence we have from research now points to *a longer life for them* as well for those who choose wisely...

We've Got Our Priorities All "Screwed Up" in Physical Activity Education and in Competitive Sport!

To many people what I have to say here will mark me as a "mean old man and a spoilsport," a grinch! However, the past few months have absolutely convinced me that we—in the developed (!) world—have our priorities all screwed up in relation to competitive sport and physical activity education. Frankly, I am so sick of "gold–medals–this" and "own–the–podium that" that I feel completely frustrated by the money, time, and attention devoted to these activities for the "minute few"! Then, on top of the Olympics Games, we also have the Paralympic Games and the Special Olympics. (Fortunately, the latter two are more like what the "big one" ought to be!) All in all, however, "enuf already..."

Please don't misunderstand me. I believe physical activity education and sport competition are wonderful activities for all people of all ages and conditions throughout their lives. There is evidence that such activity will enable people to live healthier lives longer! However, my fundamental point is that—for the good of humankind—we must build from the ground up with all people! As matters stand now, we do a fair to poor to "nil" job of physical activity education with the *very* large majority of youth (and somewhat worse for girls!). Yet, when it comes to a minute fraction of youth–"accelerated and special"–within education and the private sector–we actually do quite well with competitive sport itself.

Think about it! Suppose we did this in *this* way with any other important subject or activity in the educational curriculum (e.g., English, science, math…)? The outcry would be so loud that all activity in our everyday world would be brought to a shrieking halt peremptorily. "How dare you do this to my son (or daughter)? He (She) has a right to the same advantages that all others get! Throw the legislators, the educators, and/or any other "bum" responsible for this dereliction of duty out of office on his/her rump this very day!"

Somehow the cart has been put in front of the horse! Unless your son and daughter is gifted in regard to his/her heritage of physical skill, he/she is a *nonentity* insofar as physical activity education is concerned and is being deprived of what could be–if properly stressed and taught–a truly important educational experience. Such an experience, if carried out well (!), would not only help him or her to learn better, but would also help to keep your child or youth healthy now and prepare him/her attitude-wise and *literally* for (hopefully!) "the long journey ahead" through life.

The folks promoting the present "upside-down" approach to physical activity education, including sport competition, for *all* youth will tell you that the present overemphasis for the few is *the* way to do it. Those "on the bottom" will be inspired by seeing "all these medals arriving on our shores". They will start working to "get there" too, they say, also. I say: "Baloney"! They'll never have a chance if the arrangement continues as it is today. This is so unless, the next thing you know, the "people in control" will convince politicians to arrange things *for all* the way they are in China. Test little children for ability early; take them from their parents and send them to specially designed schools for early training. Then watch them "get those gold medals on the podium that their country 'owns'"! Glorioski!

> Note: The logic of the above argument seems impeccable. The illogical response appears to be: "That's the way the world is. 'Em that has, gits'."

Specific Ways That America ("The West") Is "Screwing Up" Sport

Note: This subtitle was coined after reading John Tirman's *100 Ways That America Is Screwing Up the World* (NY: Harper Perennial, 2006).

The first way that America (and the rest of the world) is making a terrible mistake is in unofficially promoting the idea that *"winning" is the only thing!* It's hard to believe that Canada, for example, would go against the historic ideal of Olympism by officially establishing and supporting financially an "Own the Podium" organization. Such overemphasis of the importance of involvement in (and winning in international sport competition!) is a perfect example of sport being used for nationalistic (and economic?) purposes!

Next, as a longtime physical (activity) educator, including my service as a coach of three difference sports in two different universities over a 15-year period early on in my career, somehow it truly disturbs me that schools, colleges, and universities are spending infinitely more emphasis, including time and money, on "varsity" sport for the very few rather than spending an "equitable", appropriate amount of money on intramural, after-school sports for the overwhelming majority of children and youth. If such emphasis were to be placed on any other aspect of an educational institution's "educational offerings" for "the few" rather than for "the "overwhelming majority," there would soon be a "revolution in the streets."

Thirdly, the steady development of so-called "TV Universities" in America couldn't help but debase the whole idea of "higher" education in those institutions involved. The men and women involved in competition in these universities are nothing more than semi-professional athletes hired to publicize what a "great university" they represent for whatever "notoriety" that may bring the institution so designated.

Next the whole idea of offering "athletic" scholarships where there is no proven financial need makes a mockery of the university involved unless similar "scholarships" to young people who have demonstrated ability and potential is the other aspects of life and living such as music, art, drama, communication et al. that contribute to the overall cultural development of society.

Another aspect of sport that is truly troubling to me has been the steady addition of so-called "violent" sports. I am thinking of all of those activities "where "life and limb" are threatened unnecessarily. I confess there is a personal connotation here for me too. In my sophomore year in college, I had just been elevated to the varsity football team as a fullback due to the injury of the upperclassman playing regularly in that position. Three days later scrimmaging in the mud against the freshman team, I had a most serious knee injury that required immediate surgery. However, due to inadequate (no!) medical treatment, I ended up in the college infirmary with no x-ray ever taken. This put an end to any future football or track aspirations I may have had.

Of course, this could simply be an everyday occurrence in high schools in North America today. Such inadequacy is bad enough, but what I am really referring to here is the variety of activities that have emerged and are perennially sponsored that are literally death-defying. I am thinking, for example, of the leaps. somersaults, and twists involved in winter-sport competitions and the stunts performed in figure skating and gymnastics. And how about permitting a child to sail around the world in a small sail boat by herself! I believe much of this increasingly violent and/or dangerous innovation has reached the "ridiculous" stage!

To this point, of course, I have limited the discussion to the possibility of severe injury and death in sport competition, but there's another aspects that deserves serious consideration as well. All my life I thought that the main reason for participation in sport by children and youth, in addition to wholesome, healthy experience, was that such involvement promoted the development of such qualities as fair play, honesty, and sportsmanship. However, what do we learn most recently in the history of competitive sport's "development"? *What's really important is that sport promote the development of socio-instrumental or material values.* (In Canada, for example, it's so important that Canada has made specific plans to "Own the Podium"!)

In addition, just what has happened in much of higher education in America? We now have created a situation in competitive sport in higher education where studies have shown that fair play, honesty, and sportsmanship have declined steadily throughout the athlete's four-year, university experience.

Further, the "tone" of the "athletic experience" appears to have undergone a transformation as well. I don't recall the whole idea of "trash talk" in competitive sport being so ever-present and absolutely derogatory and disgusting. Frankly, it appalls me! Still further, athletes "showboating" after specific accomplishments is unsportsmanlike and obnoxious in my opinion

Still further, society permits the probability of lifelong brain damage in professional boxing where the opponent's head is the primary target. I could sanction amateur boxing in sporting situations where there is adequate protection with headgear in a supervised situation. However, the main emphasis in so-called combative sport should be on self-defense. Amateur wrestling for both men and women is a much better, safer form of activity.

Moreover, I won't spend any words on that disgusting travesty known as "professional" wrestling featured on television, or on the more recent aberration permitting practically all-out combat known as "Extreme Sport". The latter is to me only a contradiction in terms and should be banned!

Another terrible problem that has confronted sport, of course, is the entire issue of drugs and doping in sport, an abuse that is "killing it" worldwide. Reading the daily output of the Canadian Center for Ethics in Sport on the Internet is an enlightening, but also frightening experience for me five times a week. (You are urged to google <www.cces.ca> to see first hand the excellent reports [Mon-Fri.] I am referring to...)

If all of the above isn't bad enough, to top it off the leading professional athletes on various "spectator sports" are typically receiving ridiculously high salaries based on extended-year contracts. This has the effect of creating a false sense of value on the minds of youth observing this practice. (I'm thinjking specifically of young Blacks in America in regard to basketball especially.) This is a highly important matter about which intelligent, influential people must become increasingly concerned. Competitive sport is becoming an increasingly important social force in the world, exerting almost too great an influence if this is possible. We simply cannot continue to look the other way at this problem.

Further, culture heroes are truly hard to come by these days. If we really want America and Canada to be among the finest of nations in all regards, and if we really feel that sport has an important contribution to make to the development of such a society, I believe it is time to give the highest reward and acclaim to whose who demonstrate through sport *both* a high degree of athletic ability *and* the finest of personality and character traits.

I can only conclude that times are indeed changing—for the worse. Whereas at various times throughout history, the world had its Hercules, Samson, Beowulf, and Siegfried, it was concluded in Western culture that Babe Ruth in America and Sylvester Stallone (depIcting Rocky or Rambo?) served to reinforce our conception of the ideal heroes who emerged in recent years. For example, Arnold Schwarzenegger, "the Terminator" and then former governor of California, couldn't take time off from body-building training to attend his father's funeral. These folk follow squarely in the footsteps of John Wayne and Clint Eastwood, "heroes" who display much of the same rugged, macho individualism as the old heroes of movie Westerns.

People need to understand through use of their own rational powers that they are being increasingly lured and marketed daily by others into reactions dominated more by emotions than reason. It may well be necessary to reinforce individual ego at the various geographic and social levels (i.e. community, region, state or province, and nation) by the creation of heroes and heroines in the various aspects of social living (including sport). To what extent this should be done through the artificial creation of such monstrosities as Superman, Wonderwoman, and Spiderman in one form or another, is debatable.

Further, if this type of aggrandizement (self- or promoter-sponsored) is what is happening in competitive sport, we might ask to what extent highly competitive sport is indeed a "socially useful servant" today? We don't seem to appreciate how difficult it is to make a case for the building of desirable character and personality traits through the medium of sport. Our values often seem to have become so perverted that we *condone* certain unsportsmanlike and illegal actions in sport and athletics at any level because it "excites us."

My only conclusion is that by permitting the concept of true "hero" to be applied to professional athletes unworthy of such ascription thereby unduly influencing youth as to what's important in life, is a practice that must be assiduously criticized and avoided to the greatest extent possible! Unless we do so, we are further fostering a way of life that encourages "spectatoritis" instead of actual ongoing involvement in healthful physical activity and sport that develops positive character traits.

Still further, and finally, I castigate a plan afoot now by some in Canada, for example, to place even more emphasis on competitive sport in schools. Why, pray tell. So as to do better in the Olympics! As explained above, we have now created in North America a situation where a tiny percentage of students receive attention from their teacher/coaches to develop their sport skills for the "greater glory" of their school and country This means increasingly that a teacher/coach's time is taken away from the creation of a physical activity education program (with related health information) for the large majority of "normal" youth and "special-needs" boys and girls. I state again: *Such a situation exists with no other subject-matter or activity in school systems!*

On a final note under this section of Part IV seeking to characterize some of the ways that America is "screwing up" sport, I will simply leave you, my reader, with a news release appearing in *The New York Times* (January 20, 2011). The tale that comes from "deep down" in Texas titled "A 60 Million Palace for Texas High School Football." It seems that the good citizens of Allen, Texas have decided that such a stadium had "Numero Uno" priority for their young men who aspired to greatness on the gridiron. I can come to no other conclusion but that indeed—without a doubt—history is being made!

Specific Ways That America ("The West") Is "Screwing Up" Physical Activity Education

While "varsity sport for the few proceeds merrily long," physical activity education and related health and safety education for the large majority of children and youth, including special-needs students, struggles along as a *distinctly* lesser aspect of the educational curriculum.

As one elementary school principal affiliated with PHE Canada put it succinctly when asked to assess the situation:

> "1. The pyramid is upside down. We have the majority of our specialists are teaching at the high school level (for personal reasons and coaching opportunities) instead of at the elementary level. As a result, we are losing the opportunity at the active start and early development years i.e importance of physical literacy and the learning of FMS

2. Teachers are not equipped with the tools, nor are they getting the support, to provide QDPE programs. Many of the districts have eliminated the support position at the district level.

3. Lack of funding. Many gyms and schools are not equipped with updated resources to support QDPE programs.

4. Accountability. There is minimal accountability in comparison to numeracy and literacy."

In an informal survey of some 20 men and women related closely to physical education carried out early in 2011, the following are some of the evaluations of the prevailing situation offered for consideration:

"The hours spent on 'electronic gadgetry' and in front of tv leads one to think that the concerns about obesity are being paid lip service."

"For me, the most obvious problem is that we consider sport instrumental to a number of other goals. In our current society where everything is competitive, fast-paced, and underpinned by a win-at-all-costs mentality, it's easy to see why sport replicates these values."

"It seems that we've lost the ability to see movement of the body as a pleasure in and of itself. That is, recreational sport (for "fun"), or just simply forms of "play" in sport seem to be lost. Instead, it becomes about structure, rigidity, and disciplining oneself as characteristics of good athletes that gets privileged. Kids don't just get to have fun anymore; they get pushed into sport."

"In Canada, the government has, for the past 30-40 years of sport development, maintained what Bruce Kidd called a "philosophy of excellence". The current sport development initiatives grounded in Canadian Sport for Life (CS4L) linked to Long Term Athlete Development (LTAD) state that it is a mass participation sporting model designed to encourage lifelong participation. It is **not!** LTAD is an elite model that channels youth into sport for elite purposes; it works to enhance and maximize **PERFORMANCE**, not **PARTICIPATION**."

"I think one of the most fundamental issues to the deficiencies in physical activity goes back to the industrial age influence of thinking about the mind/body dualism.... what I mean is that at a very young age we sit to learn/learn to sit. There is no doubt that this 'mind' privileging has lead to exceptional ingenuities, from steam engines to microchips, but I argue that it has done so at a cost. We no longer know ourselves in relation to the world, to each other, and to ourselves. We have over the last century come to recognize this, as our health has quickly deteriorated, and we have tried to implement ways to rectify this by publishing recommended physical activity levels... but this is still thinking with the 'head'."

"I think one of the most fundamental issues to the deficiencies in physical activity goes back to the industrial influence of thinking about the mind/body dualism. What I mean is that at a very young age we sit to learn/learn to sit. There is no doubt that this 'mind'-privileging has lead to exceptional ingenuities, from steam engines to microchips, but I argue that it has done so at a cost. We no longer know ourselves in relation to the world, to each other, and to ourselves. We have over the last century come to recognize this, as our health has quickly deteriorated, and we have tried to implement ways to rectify this by publishing recommended physical activity levels... but this is still thinking with the 'head.'"

"Several years ago we received a sizable grant here to work with overweight kids. The program lasted for several years but then collapsed. In talking with the people in charge, they said it was not the kids but the parents. They simply were not concerned about their kids' weight nor their activity level. I suspect that it is even worse now with kids spending more and more on things like computer games, constantly texting, playing computer games, etc."

"I really think that to get people of any or all ages active, we need to stop preaching about obesity "blah-blah-blah" and come up with creative ways of letting individuals young and old find the "portal" that will lead them to an active lifestyle. I did not start because I wanted to be fit, etc., I entered through the "emotional" portal. I wanted to give something to those kids in HS so I had to look or at least play the part of a role model and that meant being active. Today kids and adults need more than "eat your carrots, they are good for you". That is why I suggest helping people find their entry point to an active lifestyle."

To summarize what I have designated as the "missing links" in physical activity education at the elementary and secondary levels in public education, it appears that the following conditions prevail:

1. The best-qualified teachers are not available at the elementary level.
2. The program envisioned at the elementary level is woefully inadequate. (For example, individually oriented physical education classes should be made available for academic credit for those students interested in "personal fitness", not team sports.)
3. Schools and gymnasiums don't have updated resources.
4. Expectations for physical activity education program results, and related health and safety education are at a low level.
5. A tendency is developing to promote fitness in the community environment because schools are not "doing the job,"
6, Teachers are paid to teach, not coach; yet, too much time and energy is devoted to the latter. Hence, it is time for physical activity education teachers to teach only (i.e., not coach!).
7. There is not enough emphasis on bodily movement just for fun...
8. Parents are not setting a good example for children and youth.
9. Wholesome physical activity is not part of ideal education of the "whole person".

In summary, the various professional associations in America are doing their best to le1ad the way with guidelines and "exhortation," and it is true that new guidelines have just been issued by the Canadian government as well.

For example, an hour a day of physical activity for children and youth daily is recommended. However each state and province is its own "lord and master", and there is no directive delineation as to whom will provide the leadership, supervision, and facilities to make these guidelines "become reality." We in the field stress the need for physical activity as a basically important idea, but then the school day is typically characterized by semi-mobility–and now advancing technology has made the situation only worse!

How Should Society Solve a Serious Problem

Assuming that we are indeed confronted by a problem that has such serious ramifications for our future, what can be done? If these conditions are true, it means that we should assess the evolving situation carefully and then proceed to institute the appropriate remedies to the extent possible.

To provide us with an approach that should help to communicate with policy makers at all levels about this ever- increasing problem, *I decided to initially only offer an outline at this point that consists of a five–question approach to the building of effective communication skills recommended by Mark Bowden, a communications specialist (National Post, Canada 2008 11 24, FP3).* Subsequently, in Chapter IX titled "How Exactly Do We Get There?" I will go into considerable detail in an attempt to recommend to society how it should solve this most serious problem it is facing.

The recommended five questions to be asked are as follows:

Question 1: Where are we now?
Question 2. Why are we here?
Question 3. Where should we want to be?
Question 4. How do we get there?
Question 5. What exactly should we do?

Without attempting to enumerate specifically where any stumbling blocks might loom in our path, the field of physical activity education should keep in mind the four major processes proposed by March and Simon (*The future of human resource management*, 1958, pp. 129-131). They could be employed chronologically, as the field seeks to realize its desired immediate objectives and long-range goal. These four major processes to be followed in the achievement of the desired objectives and goals for the field are as follows:

<u>1. Problem-solving:</u>
<u>2. Persuasion:</u>
<u>3. Bargaining:</u>
<u>4. Politicking:</u>

Children and Youth Need Understanding of, and Experience With, Selected Competencies

Specifically, the child and young person needs experience in, and understanding of,

School health and safety education has grown to be so complicated that it has its own curriculum, but it should be "interwoven" with physical activity education where appropriate nevertheless.

Unless regular education can provide *all* students (i.e., special, normal, and accelerated) with the above, I do not believe a school should have a varsity athletics program for both sexes. (Only in the United States, Canada, and Japan do schools sponsor varsity teams. Typically there are outside (individual) sport clubs.) in the public sector.

> Note: It would be nice to have "varsity sport" "inside" (i.e., school spirit, etc.), but experience has shown that the physical activity and health-related education program for 95% of the students suffers where this has taken place. That's one of the reasons why we have this "sad situation" today. Hence, I've come to believe that the physical & health education teachers should *not* be coaches.
> If there is a quality program of physical education and health-related program, these teachers do not have the time and energy to be so involved...

The Public's Conception of 'Physical Education'

In 2008 the *Vancouver Sun* published a piece titled Kids' fat: Getting rid of it! (June 26, 2008). In response, I wrote "The Editors" stating that "Your headline 'kicks physical (activity) education in the teeth' on the matter of 'kids' fat' because you decided to tell the public that 'PHYS-ED WON'T CUT...' The end result of your piece was to point the public, including parents, that 'obesity and being overweight' had nothing to do with time spent in physical education classes."

However, in the Harris Report quoted, the Sun's neglected to stress that "there are improvements in bone mineral density, aerobic capacity, reduced blood pressure, and increased flexibility."
Further, how much actual physical-activity-education time are we talking about here? To a large degree the fat problem boils down to "intake versus output."

The issue here is to encourage and teach children and youth ro acquire the necessary physical interest and health education knowledge and skills. If this is done properly, they will develop a "lifestyle attitude" that encourages them to, and show them how, to "get involved." As a lifelong professional in the field in my 92nd year, I still work out every day despite arthritis and tendinitis, etc. I understand fully that, if I don't have an attitude that motivates me to "move it," I will "lose it!"

I read recently about radical reform in physical education in the European Union. We in North America have dug ourselves into a really deep hole relative to the entire disciplinary-professional controversy in the field. Looking back we who were working in the field were not able to "enlarge" the concept of 'physical education' down through the twentieth century so that people saw it as anything other except dull and repetitive activity that takes place in a school gymnasium in a school. I did say that I have also been fearful of the use of the term "kinesiology" to describe the field. I did so because using the Greek word as terminology is confusing. However, it may well be appropriate to use it at the university level as a disciplinary term—and it does avoid use of the term "physical education" that is actually a misnomer and somehow makes scholars and scientists in the field feel ashamed… If we do call ourselves "kinesiologists" when we work at the university level, we must insure that we are turning out graduates who understand kinematic movement fully, not just superficially as has been the case with typical physical education graduates…

Concluding Statement

In concluding this discussion of the status of required physical (activity) education and elective competitive sport, the overriding problem in North America today is that the United States, and Canada to a somewhat lesser degree—as supposedly democratic countries—have got their approach backwards in regard to a program of *required* physical activity education and *elective* sport for elementary and secondary education backwards!

Whatever "bona fide" *educational* experiences are "out there" should be made available to *all* children and youth. In addition, these experiences deemed essential for "the healthiest life" in a democracy should be mandated regularly up through high school graduation for all to the extent that each person is capable of being involved. There should be an irreducible minimum for all! This means that *all* should have a required, regular, excellent, graduated program of physical activity education—including related health & safety education—year after year up to high school graduation. Qualified, full-time teacher/coaches should be available to provide these educational experiences through appropriate funding.

While these basic health and fitness needs are met, if funding can be made available, *all* children and youth should be able to also choose to get involved with a variety of (1) sporting, (2) social, (3) communicative, (4) aesthetic & creative, and (5) "learning" recreational interests. Whether these additional opportunities are made available through public education or public recreation should make no difference theoretically.

Additionally, if "government" chooses to get involved in the promotion of any of these additional, after-school educational-recreational experience for youth, that's fine. However, this should take place *only if* the required curriculum needs listed above *for all* have been satisfactorily met!!! If parents are in a position financially to provide additional experiences for their offspring in after-school time, and wish to do so, this is an additional possibility, of course.

"Excellence" should be the goal in anything children and youth do, but such achievement in competitive activities should come "from the ground-up", *not* from a "top down, own the podium, subsidizing mentality" anxious to characterize one nation as superior while proving its citizens are The Greatest!"!

Moral, non-material values should come first as a result of the experience. Socio-instrumental, material values should be lesser and incidental in such experience. Competitive sport at its finest should be employed to promote the wellbeing and health of the citizens of a nation! The prevailing "unhealthy" situation must be reversed in the years ahead so that required physical activity education and elective sport competition can serve humankind in the finest way.

PART V
What Happened With Sport
and
Physical Activity Education Historically?

Primitive and Preliterate Societies

In primitive society, starting back about 50,000 years ago, there was probably very little organized purposive instruction in sport, exercise, and related expressive movement. Any incidental education was usually a byproduct of daily experience. The usual activities of labor, searching for food, rhythmic activities, and games were essential to the development of superior bodies. Physical education activities, in addition to promoting physical efficiency, helped to strengthen membership in the society and served also as a means of recreation. Mimetic games were undoubtedly drawn from life's daily activities. Sporting activities were playful and yet competitive requiring skillful movement in the pursuit of excellence. Such activity served as the precursor for later team ball games and individual activities demonstrating physical skill and endurance. Interestingly, sporting activities were often held in conjunction with religious ceremonies (often with dance movement involved as well).

China

In the ancient Chinese civilization, formal physical training and organized sport had little if any place in a culture whose major aim was to preserve and perpetuate a traditional social order. At first no strong military motive existed, although physical training was used sporadically when it did become necessary to increase military efficiency. Subsequently, in a world where Confucianism and military activity assumed greater importance, physical activity assumed greater importance. Sport and education were available to the upper classes primarily. As a type of classical education grew and various religious influences were felt, even less emphasis was placed on formal physical development, and health standards were poor indeed. In later ancient Chinese history (circa 1500 B.C.E.), the fighting arts emerged from former skills acquired in hunting. The value of training to bear arms was appreciated much more because of the changing nature of the type of combat in which the men engaged. (Interestingly, these same fighting arts became "systems" of exercise in later eras.) A great variety of team games and individual activities were carried out as well as an activity that could be termed "medical gymnastics."

India

In ancient India, the climate and religious philosophy forced a relative rejection of physical training for all save the ever-present dancing girls of the ancient world. The caste system in vogue influence sport greatly as it did all communal life. Further, those men in the military caste were trained physically to bear arms in defense of their society and were accordingly involved in sporting activities. Dancing and hatha yoga were widely practiced as well. Hatha yoga was considered to be an early stage of physical purification involving posture and breathing exercises that made the body fit for the practice of higher meditation) Harmony was sought by the freeing of "the spirit" from the material world. Typically, various hygienic rules and ritualistic dances were common to the Hindus, but were connected with religious ceremonies.

Egypt

In early Egypt also, physical training was not part of the typical educational system, although as in the other early cultures the average person, male or female, did receive a greater or lesser amount of exercise depending upon his or her daily work regimen. As the social life grew in complexity and a class structure developed, the upper class received a level of education that was not available to the great majority of people. Sports, games, and dancing were popular with the nobility, the latter activity being included in religious life for common people as well.

Sumeria (Babylon and Assyria)

The Tigris-Euphrates civilization did not seem to give physical education much status either, except for the perennial warrior class and for those occupations that demanded varying levels of physical fitness for their adequate execution. People in this culture were committed to the practical, mercantile pursuits of daily life and evidently this used up most of the energy they had to expend in their daily lives. Hittite sport evidently didn't digress much from that of the Assyrians (i.e., largely military in nature and competitive). Sporting involvement evidently wasn't necessary for human fulfillment in either culture.**Israel**

The Hebrews promoted certain physical activities and hygienic practices mainly because of the influence of their religious heritage and their desire to preserve their national unity, but it may not be assumed that they valued highly sporting activities and physical education for all. For those men involved with military affairs, it was a different story with a great variety of related activities. However, Hebrews were concerned with the health and related hygiene of all of their citizens. Later, under the influence of the Greeks and then the Romans, their attitude changed in certain locales. However, sports were never popular among *all* Hebrews of the ancient world.

Persia

In contrast, the Persians rivaled ancient Greece in many of its methods of physical training. Physical fitness was very valuable to them because it served to produce the stamina needed for great armies. They went to extremes in developing excellent hunters, horsemen, and warriors. Fencing, archery, and and discus and javelin throwing were popular, and a type of polo developed because of their ability at horse riding. However, their concept of physical education was very narrow because of their desire for military supremacy.

Greece

Physical education and athletic games were valued very highly in ancient Greek society. The Minoan culture on Crete, as well as the Mycenaean culture on the mainland, both older proto-Greek cultures, were undoubtedly strong influence in Greece's early development. The Dorian migration circa 1200 B.C.E. brought the Greeks to this peninsula. From 1100 to 700 B.C.E., the Homeric Age, athletic games held a prominent place. Local athletic festivals sprung up around markets, theaters and temples. The most notable of these was the Panathenea in Athens honoring the goddess that included similar events to the national festival that featured musical, dancing, and sporting activities that developed originally from religious ceremonies. There were several national athletic festivals, notably the Olympic Games. The aim of physical education was to produce a man of action, and great concern was shown for individual excellence. The well-rounded man-citizen-soldier was the ideal, a person who steadily increased in wisdom as well. The *Spartan* Greeks were almost completely concerned with the development of devoted citizens and outstanding soldiers or warriors.

They placed great stress upon almost unbelievably difficult physical training and hardship as part of the training at arms; the end product was an almost invincible soldier in single combat. Athletics were not considered important unless they contributed directly to soldierly prowess.

Athenian Greeks. The free citizens of Athens valued a well-round physical education program most highly for its contribution to the development of the ideal individual. However, the harmonious development of body and soul (mind) was of paramount concern. Although such overall development was available only to free men in a society where slaves were ordinarily obtained and then kept because of military victories, there has probably never been another culture—if this city-state may be so designated—in which the development of the all-round citizen was more cherished. Greek education, religion, and art influenced sport, as did sport in return influence these basic aspects of the culture. Classical Greek sport was in accord with the ideal of Hellenism, a stance that has been striven for since. Yet there were concerns about excesses creeping into the programs. In later Athenian Greece, as the society became more complex and then was conquered by Rome, gradually increasing emphasis was placed on intellectual excellence. The majority of youth lost interest in excellent physical development, and eventually extreme professionalism in athletics grew to such an extent that the former ideal was lost forever.

Rome

The Romans were much more utilitarian in their attitude toward physical training; they simply did not grasp the concept of the Greek ideal. They valued physical training for very basic reasons: it developed a man's knowledge in the skills of war, and it kept him healthy because of the strict regimen required. It helped to give a man strength and endurance and made him courageous in the process. Roman boys became involved in military camps at an early age and then remained in military service until middle age. Later in Roman history as the army became more specialized, the value of physical training for all became less apparent, although it was still practiced by most citizens to a degree for the maintenance of health and for recreational pursuits. Adults had the benefits of physical recreation through the communal baths (thermae) that evolved in Roman life providing a variety of features (e.g., exercise rooms and pools, eating facilities, and even art galleries and libraries. Athletic festivals, both those inherited from Greece and those developed on their own, thrived, but the emphasis was less on sporting events than those that provided entertainment. Fierce games in the arena, often of a highly barbaric nature involving combat with animals, were held regularly for the entertainment of the masses in order to gain political support for the various, extant office holders. In later Roman history the Olympic Games were abolished, as were the festivals and many gymnasia because of excesses that occurred.

Visigoths

The Visigoths ["visi" means east] began their successful invasions to the south about 376 C.E., and the end of the Roman Empire has usually been designated as 100 years later (476 C.E..). The period following has been commonly called, but now seemingly incorrectly thought of as, the "Dark Ages," a time when most literature and learning came to a standstill and might have been completely lost save for the newly organized monasteries. "Ill blows the wind that profits nobody" is a proverb that applies to this era. The Visigoths did possess abundant energy and splendid bodies and are presumed to have helped the virility of the civilized world of the West at that time. The Moslem leader Tarik ended the Visigothic kingdom in 711 C.E. in the battle at Guadalete.

As the immoral society of the declining Romans became a mere memory, Christianity continued to spread because of the energy, enthusiasm, and high moral standards of its followers. The Church somehow managed to survive the invasion of the barbarians and gradually became an important influence in the culture. Its continued growth seemed a certainty. Although the historic Jesus Christ in many ways was said to be anything but an ascetic, the early Christians perverted history to a degree as they envisioned the humankind's moral regeneration as the highest goal. In the process they became most concerned with their "souls" and the question of possible eternal happiness. (It should be pointed out that with the Greeks it was a mind (soul) and body dichotomy, but then St. Thomas Aquinas later added the dimension of soul or spirit to the mind and body dichotomy and made the human a "tripartite creature.") Matters of the body were presumed to be of this world, and consequently of Satan; affairs of the soul were of God.

The belief has prevailed that most churchmen were opposed to the idea of physical training, but this was subsequently called "The Great Protestant Legend" (Ballou, 1965). On balance it seems more logical that these Christians would not be opposed to the idea of hard work and strenuous physical activity, but that they would indeed be violently opposed to all types of sports, games, and athletic festivals associated with earlier pagan religions and the horrible excesses of the Roman arena and hippodrome.

And so it was that for hundreds of years during the period known as the Early Middle Ages, physical education, as known today, found almost no place within the meager educational pattern that prevailed. It was a very sterile period indeed for those interested in the promulgation of sport and physical activity of the finest type. Eventually even much of the physical labor in the fields and around the grounds of the monasteries was transferred to non-clerics. Thus, even this basic physical fitness was lost to this group as more intellectual pursuits became the rule. As is so often the case, the pendulum had swung too far in the other direction.

The Early Middle Ages (in *the West*)

Physical training was revived to a degree in the period known as The Early Middle Ages (or The Age of Chivalry). Feudal society was divided into three classes: (1) the masses, who had to work to support the other classes and to eke out a bare subsistence for themselves; (2) the clergy, who carried on the affairs of the Church; and (3) the nobles, who were responsible for the government of certain lands and territories under a king, and who also performed military duties.

During this time a physical and military education of a most strenuous type was necessary along with a required training in social conduct for the knight who was pledged to serve (1) his feudal lord, (2) the Church, and, presumably, (3) all women as well as his own lady in particular. Such an ideal was undoubtedly better in theory than in practice, but it did serve to set standards higher than those which existed previously. The aim of physical training was certainly narrow according to today's ideal, and understandably health standards were typically very poor. The Greek ideal had been forgotten, and physical education once again served a most practical objective: to produce a well-trained individual in the art of hand-to-hand combat with all of the necessary physical attributes such as strength, endurance, agility, and coordination. With the subsequent invention of machinery of war, the enemy was not always met at close range. As a result, death in battle became to a larger extent accidental and was not necessarily the result of physical weakness and ineptitude in warfare techniques. Naturally, some divergence took place in the aims and methods of military training and allied physical training.

Sporting and physical-recreational activities was limited to that which took place in schools located in palaces, monastic schools, and cathedrals–and in tournaments associated with chivalry. Some festivals encouraged sport (e.g., the Tailteann Games and the Fair of Carman in Ireland). Various ball games (e.g. several similar to field hockey and rugby) were played.

In the educational system of the Early Middle Ages prior to the Renaissance period of the later Middle Ages, there were four approaches designated as (1) monasticism, (2) scholasticism, (3) chivalry, and (4) the guild system (Van Dalen, Mitchell, and Bennett, 1953). Chivalry can be classified as social education of an aristocratic nature (as opposed to democratic) nature that included military, physical, and religious-moral training. Physical education was not included in the Seven Liberal Arts of what was called higher education.

To summarize the training that occurred in sporting, military, and basic physical activity of the Early Middle Ages, the following points may be made: (1) the presumed negative outlook of the Church against *all* physical activity has been overemphasized; (2) there is some evidence that physical fitness was maintained in Western monasteries through manual labor; (3) physical training was revived strongly during the Age of Chivalry; (4) the physical fitness of farmers (according to the military standards of the time at any rate) was not very high, and their physical recreation patterns were inadequate because of their low social status, and (5) the educational system of the burghers in the developing towns and cities did not provide regular physical training, but did develop a pattern of modified physical recreation— characterized by space limitations—that contributed to overall social goals of the time.

The "'Middle-Ages' approach" followed by Van Dalen *et al.* for their analysis of "physical education for the medieval disciplines" divided the entire medieval period of the Middle Ages into four chronologically overlapping "approaches" to physical education: (1) physical education for early Christian education, (2) physical education for moral discipline, (3) physical education for social discipline (in feudal society), and (4) physical education for vocational discipline of the new middle class. Just before the Renaissance, a transitional period occurred, accompanied by a decline of feudalism and a rise in nationalism. With more vigorous trade and community growth, a stronger middle class gradually arose, with a resultant demand for an improved educational system designed to prepare the young male for his lifetime occupation. Informal physical exercise and games contributed to the social and recreational goals of the young townspeople. Such physical activity also enhanced military training. It is interesting to note, also, that games and informal sports were accompanying features of the frequent religious holidays.

The Later Middle Ages *(in the West)*

The period following feudalism was known as The Later Middle Ages (or The Renaissance). At this time it was natural that learned people should begin to look back to the periods in history that were characterized by even roughly similar societies. The Church was solidly entrenched, and there was much enthusiasm for scholarship in the fields of law, theology, and medicine. Understandably this scholasticism and emphasis on intellectual discipline found little if any room for physical education. Unorganized sports and games were the only activities of this nature in either the cathedral schools pr in the universities that had been established relatively recently.

In the late 14th and in the 15th century, however, a type of humanism developed that stressed the worth of the individual—and once again the physical side of the person was considered. Most of the humanistic educators appreciated the earlier Greek ideal and emphasized the care and proper development of the body. Vittorino da Feltre set an example for others in his school at the court of the Prince of Mantua in northern Italy. One of his aims was to discipline the body so hardship might be endured with the least possible hazard. His pupils were some day to bear arms and had to know the art of warfare. Individual and group sports and games were included because of the "recreative" nature of such activity. Da Feltre believed that the ability of a youth to learn in the classroom depended to a considerable extent upon the physical condition of the individual, a belief for which there is some evidence today.

A significant advancement in the eyes of many was the restoration of the ideal that there should be a balance among the various aspects of the educational curriculum. The Renaissance world eventually realized that the world had indeed known a much better type of education at the height of the Greek and Roman civilizations. To glean the best from the literature of these cultures, however, meant that scholars had to comprehend purer Latin and a knowledge of Greek as well. Thus began a most diligent effort to regain these "fabled treasures," an enterprise that very soon gave Latin and Greek, the classics, a central place in a largely humanities curriculum. Interestingly, the growth of a leisure class at this point meant that there would be increased time for an increased number to benefit from such knowledge and skills. Also, the interests of many of these people were of this world, not of some intangible realm.

This new *humanistic* curriculum included intellectual, esthetic, moral, and physical-activity aspects. Humans were once again presented with ideal that stressed a well-balanced education, one that even included aspects of the etiquette of the former era. It must be noted, however, that there was a variety of emphases with this "new" approach. The esthetic aspects were stressed more in southern Europe, while moral education received greater attention in the north. Stylistic elegance counted for more in Italy than in Germany. In the latter instance educators placed greater emphasis on what they felt was a more "discriminating" mind.

One famous humanist school in Italy was led by Vittorino da Feltre at the court of the Duke of Mantua. Another humanist, Erasmus from Holland, sought change from within the Catholic church and had a strong influence on European education after 1500. Although the humanistic ideal was eventually debased, it did have an enormous influence on the education of the elite during the Renaissance period. The classics became firmly entrenched in the school curriculum and had to be mastered prior to university education. Further, to a degree, the educational aim was broadened to the extent that preparation for service in life, whether as a nobleman, priest, merchant, or politician, received due emphasis.

In retrospect, it was natural that learned people during the Renaissance should begin to look back to the periods in history that were characterized by even roughly similar societies. The Church was still solidly entrenched, of course, and there was much enthusiasm for scholarship in the fields of law, theology, and medicine. Understandably this scholasticism with its emphasis on intellectual discipline found little if any room for physical education. Unorganized sports and games were the only activities of this nature in the cathedral schools and in the universities that had been established relatively recently.

Early Modern Period

In what has been called the Early Modern Period, there followed a decline in liberal education as the schools lost their original aim and began the study of the languages of Greece and Rome exclusively while unfortunately neglecting the other aspects of these civilizations. The importance of physical training for youth again declined, even as preparation for life work was crowded out for many by preparation for university education. Thus, when the spirit of Italian humanistic education reached into Europe, the Greek ideal of physical education and sporting activity was realized by only a relatively few individuals. Those involved with the Protestant Reformation did practically nothing to encourage physical education activities with the possible exception of Martin Luther himself, who had an interest in wrestling and who evidently realized a need for the physical training of youth. Some educators rebelled against the narrow type of education that had come into vogue, but they were the exception rather than the rule.

For example, Rabelais satirized the education of the time in his depiction of the poor results of the typical Latin grammar school graduate. His Gargantua was a "dolt and blockhead," but subsequently became a worthwhile person when his education became more well-rounded. Also, Michel de Montaigne, the great French essayist of the 16th century, believed that the education of the person should not be dichotomized into the typical mind-body approach. Further, other educators such as Locke, Mulcaster, and Comenius recognized the value of physical exercise. Some educational leaders in the 17th century stressed character development as the primary educational aim, but a number of them believed also in the underlying need for health and physical fitness. John Locke, for example, even stressed the importance of recreation for youth. However, his ideas were far from being accepted as the ideal for all in a society characterized by a variety of social classes.

The Age of Enlightenment

The 18th century in Europe was a period of change as to what might be called more modern political, social, and educational ideals. In France, Voltaire denounced both the Church and the state. Rousseau decried the state of society also, as well as the condition of education in this period. He appeared to desire equality for all and blamed the civilization of the time for the unhappiness in the world. He urged the adoption of a "back to nature" movement, because it seemed to him that everything had degenerated under the influence of what we have come to call organized society.

In his heralded educational treatise *Emile*, he described what he considered to be the ideal education for a boy. From the age of one to five, he stressed, the only concern should be for the growth and physical welfare of the young person. From five to 12 years of age, the idea of *natural* growth was to be continued as the strong, healthy youngster learned about the different aspects of his environment. Rousseau did consider the person to be an indivisible entity and was firmly convinced of the need to devote attention to the developmental growth of the *entire* organism. For him it was not possible to know when an activity lost its "physical" value and began to possess so-called "intellectual" worth.

At this point in Europe's history, many strong social forces, with the opinions of such men as Voltaire and Rousseau, led to the ruination of the existing political and social structure. The reconstruction developed gradually in the 19th century concurrent with many changes, educational and otherwise, that influenced physical education directly and indirectly. For example, Johann Basedow started a naturalistic school in Dessau based on the fundamental ideas of Rousseau. This school termed "Philanthropinum", was the first in modern Europe to admit children from all social classes and to give physical education a place in the daily curriculum. A number of other prominent educators during this period expressed what they felt to be the proper place of physical training in the curriculum thereby helping to mold public opinion to a degree. Outstanding among these men were Guts Muths, Pestalozzi, and (philosopher) Immanuel Kant. Friedrich Froebel, who ranks along with Pestalozzi as a founder of modern pedagogy, offered the first planned program of education through play.

Emerging Nationalism

As it turned out, the rise of nationalism had a direct relationship to the development of physical training in modern Europe. Both the French and American revolutions sparked feelings of strong loyalty to country in many parts of the world. Gradually, politicians recognized education as a vital means of promoting the progress of developing nations. Education for citizenship, therefore, stressed the obligation of youth to develop itself fully for the glory of the nation. Historians have pointed out that nationalistic education is probably a necessary step toward subsequent internationalism, but it must be stated that still today this assertion remains to be proved "solidly." Even if so, it has often brought grief to many in the process.

Germany

The *Turnvereine* (gymnastic societies) in Germany originated during the first decade of the 19th century. Friedrich L. Jahn, a staunch patriot of the time, is considered the father of this movement. He wished fervently that his people would become strong enough to throw off the yoke of the French conquerors. Jahn believed that exercise was a vital means to employ in the ideal plan of growth and development for the individual. He held also that there was a certain mental and moral training to be derived from experience at the *Turnplatz* (the site where exercises were performed). The War of Liberation for Prussia was waged successfully in 1813, and his work undoubtedly helped the cause. *Turnen* (German gymnastics) underwent periods of popularity and disfavor during the next 40 years. Later the *Turnen* societies cautiously accepted the various games and sports of the sport movement.

Adolph Spiess did a great amount of work in planning and developing school gymnastics as he strove to have physical training included as an important part of the child's education. In 1849 he established normal classes in this type of gymnastics at Darmstadt. Since 1860 Germany has fully recognized the importance of school gymnastics, and this subject has continually grown in prominence for the pre-university years. However, what is included in the curriculum has changed markedly, even to a name change (i.e., Sport).

The military motive was very influential in shaping the development of physical training in a number of other European countries, also, with certain individual variations. Scientific advances have gradually brought about the inauguration of new theories in keeping with the advancing times.

Great Britain

Great Britain's isolated position in relation to the European continent made rigorous training for warfare and national defense less necessary and tended to foster the continuance of interest in outdoor sports. In feudal England archery was the most popular sport, but in the 15th century golf rivaled it until the king banned it by proclamation because of the disturbance it was creating. A bit later, however, golf was accepted by nobles, and the ban was lifted. Field hockey, cricket, bowling, quoits, tennis, rugby, hammer throwing, and pole vaulting had their origins in the British Isles.

Many of the other traditional sports originated elsewhere but were soon adopted by the people in England too. In the early 19th century an urgent need was felt for some type of systematized physical training. Clias, Ehrenhoff, Georgii, and Maclaren were some of the men who introduced specialized methods of physical training and culture to the British people. Any stress on systematized school gymnastics and the movement for improved health did not, however, discourage after-school sport participation in any way. Down through years since then, Great Britain has encouraged active participation by all schoolchildren and avoided the overtraining of the few.

The Modern Olympic Games

The revival of the Olympic Games in 1896 was brought about largely through the efforts of Baron Pierre de Coubertin of France. Certainly much interest has been created with the successive holding of these Games every four years in countries all over the world (except in wartime). Today considerable concern is being expressed in some quarters about the media's preoccupation with team scores and the accompanying excessive nationalistic flag-raising and the playing of national anthems. It probably can be argued that international goodwill has been fostered by this highly competitive international sport, but the "ideal of Olympism" expressed by de Coubertin and associates seems to have been largely lost in all the hoopla and excessive commercialization that has steadily increased ever since.

A cynic could argue that all of this "goodwill" resulted in two worldwide wars and innumerable sectional wars being fought since the advent of the Modern Games. However, we must give some credence to the optimist's position that it has been worthwhile to promote such athletic competition in the hope that such "friendly strife" might have some constructive influence on the development of peace and international goodwill. Throughout the 20th century, therefore, sport and games for men, and then increasingly for women, too, have become ever more popular throughout Europe and in most other parts of the world as well.

The Twentieth Century

Now that we have looked at a synopsis of the values that people have held (or haven't held!) for sport and physical education throughout history, in the context of this book it would serve no significant purpose to review the history of this subject at length for the entire world. Histories of sport and/or physical education have been made available. As it happened, the significance of play and its possibilities in the educative process were really not comprehended in any significant way anywhere until well up in the 1800s. Typically the many educational systems were opposed to the entire idea of what would be included in a fine program of sport and physical activity education today.

The United States of America

According to historian Norma Schwendener (1942), the history of physical education in the United States could be divided into four distinct periods: (1) The Colonial Period (1609-1781); (2) The Provincial Period (1781-1885); (3) The Period of the Waning of European Influence (1885-1918); and (4) The Period of American Physical Education (1918-). Although this classification will not be followed here, the reader can get some perspective from Schwendener's earlier outline, and a similar "longitudinal approach" is followed here

The Colonial Period. Living conditions in the American colonies in the 17th and 18th centuries were harsh, the finer elements of then civilized life being possible for only a relatively few wealthy individuals. The culture itself had been transported from Europe with its built-in class distinctions. The rules of primogeniture and entail served to strengthen such status. Slavery, and near-slavery, were general practice, especially in the South, and the right to vote was typically restricted to property owners. Cultural contrasts were marked. Religion was established legally. Geography, differences between the environment in the North and South, had a great deal to do with many differences that were evident. Actually, there was even considerable feeling against democratic principles both from a political and social standpoints. Any consideration of educational practice must, therefore, be viewed in the light of these conditions.

Most of the American colonies established between 1607 and 1682 were guided in their educational outlook and activities by England's contemporary practices, the influence of other European countries being negligible at first. Education was thought to be a function of the Church, not the State. By today's standards, the provisions made for education were extremely inadequate. In a pioneer country characterized by a hazardous physical environment, the settlers were engaged in a daily struggle for their very existence. Early colonists migrated into different regions relatively close to the eastern coastline almost by chance. These differing environments undoubtedly influenced the social order of the North and the South; yet, for several generations there were many points of similarity in the traditions and experiences of the people as a whole. They all possessed a common desire for freedom and security, hopes that were to be realized only after a desperate struggle.

The church was the institution through which the religious heritage, and also much of the educational heritage, was preserved and advanced. The first schools can actually be regarded as the fruits of the Protestant revolts in Europe. The settlers wanted religious freedom, but the traditionalists among them insisted that a knowledge of the Gospel was required for personal salvation. The natural outcome was the creation of schools to help children learn to read; thus, it was the dominant Protestant churches that brought about the establishment of the elementary schools.

Three types of attitude developed toward education. The first was the compulsory-maintenance attitude of the New England Puritans, who established schools by colony legislation of 1642 and 1647. The second attitude was that of the parochial school, and this was best represented by Pennsylvania where private schools were made available for those who could afford it. The pauper-school, non-State-interference attitude was the third. It was best exemplified by Virginia and the southern colonies. Many of these people had come to America for profit rather than religious freedom, the result being that they tended to continue school practice as it had existed in England. In all these schools, discipline was harsh and sometimes actually brutal. The curriculum consisted of the three R's and spelling, but the books were few and the teachers were generally unprepared.

The pattern of secondary education had been inherited from England too. In most of the colonies, and especially in New England, so-called Latin grammar schools appeared. Also, higher education was not neglected. Nine colleges were founded mainly through the philanthropy of special individuals or groups. In all of these institutions, theology formed an important part of the curriculum. A notable exception that began a bit later was the Academy and College of Philadelphia where Benjamin Franklin exerted a strong influence.

Early Games, Contests, and Exercise. What about physical training and play for the young? What were the objectives for which people strove historically in what later was called physical education in the United States? We will now take a look at the different roles that such development physical activity played (or didn't play!) in the educational pattern of the States over a period of several centuries down to the present day. This entire time period covering the history of physical education in the United States could be divided logically into four distinct periods: the Colonial Period (1609-1781); the Provincial Period (1781-1885); the Period of the Waning of European Influence (1885-1918); and the Period of American Physical Education (1918-).

Because the population of the colonial United States was mostly rural, one could not expect organized gymnastics and sports to find a place in the daily lives of the settlers. Most of the colonies, with the possible exception of the Puritans, engaged in the games and contests of their motherlands to the extent that they had free time. Even less than today, the significance of play and its possibilities in the educative process were not really comprehended; in fact, the entire educational system was opposed to the idea of what would be included in a fine program of sport and physical education today.

The 18th Century. With the advent of the 18th century, the former religious interest began to slacken. The government gradually developed more of a civil character with an accompanying tendency to create schools with a native vein or character. This was accompanied by a breakdown in some of the former aristocratic practices followed by a minority. The settled frontier expanded, new interests in trade and shipping grew, and the population increased. An evident trend toward individualism characterized this period as well. Several American industries date back to this time, the establishment of iron mills being most noteworthy.

Although the colonists were typically restricted by the financial practices placed by the English on the use of money, there was sufficient prosperity to bring about a change in the appearance of the established communities. An embryonic class structure began to form, with some colonials achieving a certain amount of social status by the holding of land and office. However, there were other concerns such as a series of small wars with the Spanish and the French extending from 1733 to 1763. These struggles were interspersed by period of cold war maneuvering. What was called the Seven Years' War (1755-1763) ended with the colonies as a fairly solid political and economic unit. However, the British method of governance over the colony was a constant source of annoyance and serious concern with the result that a strong nationalistic, separatist feeling emerging about 1775.

Beginning in the third decade of the eighteenth century, a revival of religious interest was apparent. This occasioned a recurring strong emphasis on religious education in the elementary schools. However, with the stirring of economic, political, and nationalistic forces from approximately 1750 onward, a period of relative religious tolerance resulted. This was accompanied by a broader interest in national affairs by many. The result was a lesser emphasis on the earlier religious domination of the elementary curriculum.

Secondary education was still provided by the grammar schools. These schools, generally located in every large town, were supported by the local government and by private tuition. The curricula were non-utilitarian and were designed to prepare boys for college entrance. Insofar as higher education was concerned, the pattern had been established from the beginning (Harvard College in 1636) after the European university type of liberal arts education with a strong emphasis on mental discipline and theology.

Despite the above, the reader should keep in mind that there were still very few heavily populated centers. In the main, frontier life especially, but also life in small villages, was still most rigorous. Such conditions were simply not conducive to intellectual life with high educational standards. Educational theorists had visions of a fine educational system, of course, but state constitutional provisions regarding education were very limited, and the federal constitution didn't say anything about educational standards at all. The many new social forces at work offered some promise, but with the outbreak of the War of Independence formal education came to almost a complete standstill.

The last 25 years of the 18th century saw a great many changes in the life of the United States. In the first place, many of the revolutionaries who started the war lived to tell about it and to help in the sound reconstruction of the young nation. State and federal constitutions had to be planned, written, and approved. Also, it was very important to the early success of the country that commerce be revived, a process that was accomplished sooner by the South because of the nature of the commodities they produced. New lines of business and trade were established with Russia, Sweden, and the Orient. The Federal Convention of 1787 managed to complete what has turned out to be possibly the most successful document in all of history, the Constitution of the United States of America. Then George Washington's administration began, and it was considered successful both at home and abroad. Interestingly, the concurrent French Revolution became an issue in American politics, but Washington persuaded his government to declare a position of neutrality (although he was hard pressed to maintain it).

As soon as the War of Independence in the U.S.A. was over, considerable attention was turned to education with the result that higher and secondary education improved. The colleges of the North took longer to recover from the War than those in the South where soon an imposing list of both private, religiously endowed, and state-sponsored institutions were founded.

Early Advocates of "Physical Training". At the secondary level, the institutions that succeeded the Latin grammar schools became known as the academies. Their aim was to prepare youth to meet life and its many problems, a reflection of the main influences of the Enlightenment in America. With such an emphasis, it is natural that the physical welfare of youths gradually was considered to be more important that it had been previously. Some of the early academies, such as Dummer, Andover, Exeter, and Leicester, were founded and incorporated before 1790. This movement reached its height around 1830 when there was said to be approximately 800 such schools throughout the country.

Many of the early American educators and statesmen supported the idea that both the body and the mind needed attention in our educational system. Included among this number were Benjamin Franklin, Noah Webster, Thomas Jefferson, Horace Mann, and Henry Barnard. Further support came from Captain Alden Partridge, one of the early superintendents of the United States Military Academy at West Point, who crusaded for the reform of institutions of higher education. He deplored the entire neglect of physical culture.

The 19th Century. With the stage set for the United States to enter a most important period in her history, the 19th century witnessed steady growth along with a marked increase in nationalism. There was a second war with Great Britain, the War of 1812. In the ensuing nationalist era, many political changes or "adjustments" were carried out in relations with Britain and other nations where necessary. The Monroe Doctrine declared to the world that countries in this hemisphere should be left alone to develop as they saw fit and were not to be used by outside powers for colonization. However, at home dissent was growing as the North and the South were being divided. The North was being changed by virtue of the Industrial Revolution taking place, along with many educational and humanitarian movements. The South, conversely, continued to nurture a different type of society regulated by what has been called a slave and cotton economy.

In the realm of education, the first 50 years of the new national life was a period of transition from the control of the church to that of the State. State control and support gradually seemed more feasible, although the change was seemingly slow in coming. Political equality and religious freedom, along with changing economic conditions, made education for all a necessity. By 1825, therefore, a tremendous struggle for the creation of the American State School was underway. In the field of public education, the years from 1830 to 1860 have been regarded by some educational historians "The Architectural Period."

North American Turners. In the early 19th century German gymnastics (Turnen) came to the United States through the influx of such men as Charles Beck, Charles Follen, and Francis Lieber. However, the majority of the people were simply not ready to recognize the possible values of these activities imported from foreign lands. The Turnverein movement (in the late 1840s) before the Civil War was very important for the advancement of physical training. The Turners advocated that mental and physical education should go hand in hand in the public schools. As it developed, they were leaders in the early physical education movement around 1850 in such cities as Boston, St. Louis, and Cincinnati.

In the United States, for example, it was the organized German-American Turners primarily, among certain others, who came from their native Germany and advocated that mental and physical education should proceed hand in hand in the public schools. The Turners' opposition to military training as a substitute for physical education contributed to the extremely differentiated pattern of physical education in the post-Civil War era. Their influence offset the stress on military drill in the land-grant colleges created by Congress passing the Morrill Act in the United States in 1862. The beginning of U.S.A. sport as we know it also dates to this period and, from the outset, college faculties took the position that games and sport were not a part of the basic educational program. The colleges and universities, the YMCAs, the Turners, and the proponents of the various foreign systems of gymnastics made significant contributions during the last quarter of the 19th century.

Other leaders in this period were George Barker Win(d)ship and Dioclesian Lewis. Windship was an advocate of heavy gymnastics and did much to convey the mistaken idea that great strength should be the goal of all gymnastics, as well as the notion that strength and health were completely synonymous. Lewis, who actually began the first teacher training program in physical education in the country in 1861, was a crusader in every sense of the word; he had ambitions to improve the health of all Americans through his system of light calisthenics—an approach that he felt would develop and maintain flexibility, grace, and agility as well. His stirring addresses to many professional and lay groups did much to popularize this type of gymnastics, and to convey the idea that such exercise could serve a desirable role in the lives of those who were weaker and perhaps even sickly (as well as those who were naturally stronger).

The Civil War between the North and the South wrought a tremendous change in the lives of the people. In the field of education, the idea of equality of educational opportunity had made great strides; the "educational ladder" was gradually extending upward with increasing opportunity for ever more young people. For example, the number of high schools increased fivefold between 1870 and 1890. The state was gradually assuming a position of prime importance in public education. In this process, state universities were helpful as they turned their attention to advancing the welfare of the individual states. The Southern states lagged behind the rest of the country due to the ravages of War with subsequent reconstruction, racial conflict, and continuing fairly "aristocratic theory" of education. In the North, however, President Eliot of Harvard called for education reform in 1888. One of his main points was the need for greatly improved teacher training.

After the Civil War, the Turners through their societies continued to stress the benefits of physical education within public education. Through their efforts it was possible to reach literally hundreds of thousands of people either directly or indirectly. The Turners have always opposed military training as a substitute for physical education. Further, the modern playground movement found the Turners among its strongest supporters. The Civil War had demonstrated clearly the need for a concerted effort in the areas of health, physical education, and physical recreation (not to mention competitive sports and games). The Morrill Act passed by Congress in 1862 helped create the land-grant colleges. At first, physical education as a subject-matter was not aided significantly by this development because of the stress on military drill in these institutions. All in all, the best that can be said is that an extremely differentiated pattern of physical education was present in the post-Civil War of the country.

Beginning of Organized Sport. The beginning of organized sport in the United States as we now know it dates back approximately to the Civil War period. Baseball and tennis were introduced in that order during this period and soon became very popular. Golf, bowling, swimming, basketball, and a multitude of other so-called minor sports made their appearance in the latter half of the nineteenth century. American football also started its rise to popularity at this time. The Amateur Athletic Union was organized in 1888 to provide governance for amateur sport. Unfortunately, controversy about amateurism has surrounded this organization almost constantly ever since. Nevertheless, it has given invaluable service to the promotion of that changing and often evanescent phenomenon that this group has designated as "legitimate amateur sport."

The Young Men's Christian Association. The YMCA traces its origins back to 1844 in London, England, when George Williams organized the first religious group. This organization has always stressed as one of its basic principles that physical welfare and recreation were helpful to the moral well-being of the individual. Some of the early outstanding physical education leaders in the YMCA in the United States were Robert J. Roberts, Luther Halsey Gulick, and James Huff McCurdy.

Early Physical Activity in Higher Education. It was toward the middle of the 19th century that the colleges and universities began to think seriously about the health of their students. The University of Virginia had the first real gymnasium, and Amherst College followed in 1860 with a two-story structure devoted to physical education. President Stearns urged the governing body to begin a department of physical culture in which the primary aim was to keep the student in good physical condition. Dr. Edward Hitchcock headed this department for an unprecedented period of fifty years until his death in 1911. Yale and Harvard erected gymnasiums for similar purposes in the late 1800s, but their programs were not supported adequately until the warly 1900s. These early facilities were soon followed elsewhere by the development of a variety of "exercise buildings" built along similar lines.

Harvard University was fortunate in the appointment of Dr. Dudley Allen Sargent to head its recognized Hemenway Gymnasium. This dedicated physical educator and physician led the university to a preeminent position in the field, and his program became a model for many other colleges and universities. He stressed physical education for the individual. His goal was the attainment of a perfect structure—harmony in a well-balanced development of mind and body.

From the outset, college faculties had taken the position that games and sports were not necessarily a part of the basic educational program. Interest in them was so intense, however, that the wishes of the students, while being denied, could not be thwarted. Young college men evidently strongly desired to demonstrate their abilities in the various sports against presumed rivals from other institutions. Thus, from 1850 to 1880 the rise of interest in intercollegiate sports was phenomenal. Rowing, baseball, track and field, football, and later basketball were the major sports. Unfortunately, college representatives soon found that these athletic sports needed control as evils began to creep in and partially destroy the values originally intended as goals.

An Important Decade for Physical Education. The years from 1880 to 1890 undoubtedly form one of the most important decades in the history of physical education in the United States. The colleges and universities, the YMCAs, the Turners, and the proponents of the various foreign systems of gymnastics made contributions during this brief period. The Association for the Advancement of Physical Education (now AAHPERD) was founded in 1885, with the word "American" being added the next year. This professional organization was the first of its kind in the field in the world and undoubtedly stimulated teacher education markedly. An important early project was the plan for developing a series of experiences in physical activity—called "physical education"—the objectives of which would be in accord with the existing pattern of general education. The struggle to bring about widespread adoption of such a program followed. Early legislation implementing physical education was enacted in five states before the turn of the 20th century.

The late 19th century saw the development also of the first efforts in organized recreation and camping for children living in underdeveloped areas in large cities. The first playground was begun in Boston in 1885. New York and Chicago followed suit shortly thereafter, no doubt to a certain degree as a result of the ill effects of the Industrial Revolution. This was actually the meager beginning of the present tremendous recreation movement in our country. Camping, both that begun by private individuals and organizational camping, started before the turn of the century as well; it has flourished similarly since that time and has been an important supplement to the entire movement.

Although criticism of the educational system as a whole was present between 1870 and 1890, it really assumed large scale proportions in the last decade of the 19th century. All sorts of innovations and reforms were being recommended from a variety of quarters. The social movement in education undoubtedly had a relationship to a rise in political progressivism. Even in the universities, the formalism present in psychology, philosophy, and the social sciences was coming under severe attack. Out in the public schools, a different sort of conflict was raging. Citizens were demanding that the promise of American life should be reflected through change and a broadening of the school's purposes. However, although the seeds of this educational revolution were sown in the 19th century, the story of its accomplishment belongs to the present century.

The Twemtieth Century. In the early 20th century Americans began to do some earnest thinking about their educational aims and values. Whereas the earliest aim in U.S.A. educational history had been religious in nature, this was eventually supplanted by a political aim consistent with emerging nationalism. But then an overwhelming utilitarian, economic aim seemed to overshadow the political aim. It was at this time also that the beginnings of a scientific approach to educational problems forced educators to take stock of the development based on a rationale other than the sheer increase in student enrollment.

Then there followed an effort to consider aims and objectives from a sociological orientation. For the first time, education was conceived in terms of *complete* living as a citizen in an evolving democracy. The influence of John Dewey and others encouraged the viewing of the curriculum as child-centered rather than subject-centered. Great emphasis was placed on individualistic aims with a subsequent counter demand for a theory stressing more of a social welfare orientation.

The relationship between health and physical education and the entire system of education strengthened during the first quarter of the 20th century. Many states passed legislation requiring physical education in the curriculum, especially after the damning evidence of the draft statistics in World War I (Van Dalen et al., 1953, p. 432). Simultaneous with physical education's achievement of a type of maturity through such legislation, the struggle between the inflexibility of the various foreign systems of gymnastics and the individualistic freedom of the so-called "natural movement" was being waged with increasing vigor. Actually the rising interest in sports and games soon made the conflict unequal, especially when the concept of athletics for all really began to take hold in the second and third decades of the century.

The natural movement was undoubtedly strengthened further by much of the evidence gathered by many natural and social scientists (p. 423). A certain amount of the spirit of Dewey's philosophy took hold within the educational environment, and this new philosophy and accompanying methodology and techniques began to be effective in the light of the changing ideals of the evolving democracy. Despite this pragmatic influence, however, the influence of philosophic idealism remained strong with its emphasis on the development of individual personality and the possible inculcation of moral and spiritual values through the transfer of training theory applied to sports and games.

The tempo of life in the United States seemed to increase in the 20th century. The times were indeed changing as evidenced, for example, by one devastating war after another. In retrospect there were so many wars— World War I, World War II, the Korean War, the Vietnam War, and the seemingly ever-present "cold war" after the global conflict of the 1940s. They had an inescapable, powerful influence on society along with the worldwide depression of the 1930s. Looking back on 20th century history is a frightening experience. So much has happened, and it has happened so quickly. The phenomenon of change is as ubiquitous today at the start of the 21st century as are the historic nemeses of death and taxes.

In the public realm, social legislation and political reform made truly significant changes in the lives of people despite the leavening, ever-present struggle between conservative and liberal forces. Industry and business assumed gigantic proportions, as did the regulatory controls of the federal government. The greatest experiment in political democracy in the history of the world was grinding ahead with deliberate speed, but with occasional stopping-off sessions while "breath was caught." The idealism behind such a plan that amounted to "democratic socialism" was at times being challenged from all quarters. Also, wars and financial booms and depressions (or later recessions) weren't the types of developments that made planning and execution simple matters. All of these developments mentioned above have had their influence on the subject at hand—education (and, of course, physical education and sport).

In the early 20th century, United States citizens began to do some serious thinking about their educational aims or values. The earliest aim in U.S.A. educational history had been religious in nature, an approach that was eventually supplanted by a political aim consistent with emerging nationalism. But then an overwhelming utilitarian, economic aim seemed to overshadow the political aim. The tremendous increase in high school enrollment forced a reconsideration of the aims of education at all levels of the system. Training for the elite was supplanted by an educational program to be mastered by the many. It was at this time also that the beginnings of a scientific approach to educational problems forced educators to take stock of the development based on theory and a scholarly rationale other than one forced on the school simply because of a sheer increase in numbers.

Then there followed an effort on the part of many people to consider aims and objectives from a sociological orientation. For the first time, education was conceived in terms of complete living as a citizen of an evolving democracy. The influence of John Dewey and others encouraged the viewing of the curriculum as child-centered rather than subject-centered—a rather startling attempt to alter the long-standing basic orientation that involved the rote mastery of an amalgam of educational source material. The Progressive Education Movement placed great emphasis on individualistic aims. This was subsequently countered by a demand for a theory stressing a social welfare orientation rather than one so heavily pointed to individual development.

The relationship between school health education and physical education grew extensively during the first quarter of the 20th century, and this included their liaison with the entire system of education. Health education in all its aspects was viewed seriously, especially after the evidence surfaced from the draft statistics of World War I. Many states passed legislation requiring varying amounts of time in the curriculum devoted to the teaching of physical education. National interest in sports and games grew at a phenomenal rate in an era when economic prosperity prevailed. The basis for school and community recreation was being well-laid.

Simultaneously with physical education's achievement of a type of maturity brought about legislation designed to promote physical fitness and healthy bodies, the struggle between the inflexibility of the various foreign systems of gymnastics and the individual freedom of the so-called "natural movement" was being waged with increasing vigor. Actually the rising interest in sports and games soon made the conflict unequal, especially when the concept of "athletics for all" really began to take hold in the second and third decades of the century.

Conflicting Educational Philosophies. Even today the significance of play and its possibilities in the educative process have not really been comprehended. In fact, until well up in the 1800s in the United States, the entire educational system was opposed to the entire idea of what would be included in a fine program of sport and physical education today. It was the organized German-American Turners primarily, among certain others, who came to this continent from their native Germany and advocated that mental and physical education should proceed hand in hand in the public schools. The Turners' opposition to military training as a substitute for physical education contributed to the extremely differentiated pattern of physical education in the post-Civil War era. Their influence offset the stress on military drill in the land-grant colleges created by Congress passing the Morrill Act in the United States in 1862. The beginning of U.S.A. sport as we know it also dates to this period and, from the outset, college faculties took the position that games and sport were not a part of the basic educational program. The colleges and universities, the YMCAs, the Turners, and the proponents of the various foreign systems of gymnastics all made contributions during the last quarter of the 19th century.

In the early 20th century Americans began to do some earnest thinking about their educational aims and values. Whereas the earliest aim in U.S.A. educational history had been religious in nature, this was eventually supplanted by a political aim consistent with emerging nationalism. But then an overwhelming utilitarian, economic aim seemed to overshadow the political aim. It was at this time also that the beginnings of a scientific approach to educational problems forced educators to take stock of the development based on a rationale other than the sheer increase in student enrollment.

Then there followed an effort to consider aims and objectives from a sociological orientation. For the first time, education was conceived in terms of complete living as a citizen in an evolving democracy. The influence of John Dewey and others encouraged the viewing of the curriculum as child-centered rather than subject-centered. Great emphasis was placed on individualistic aims with a subsequent counter demand for a theory stressing more of a social welfare orientation.

The relationship between health and physical education and the entire system of education strengthened during the first quarter of the 20th century. Many states passed legislation requiring physical education in the curriculum, especially after the damning evidence of the draft statistics in World War I (Van Dalen, Bennett, and Mitchell, 1953, p. 432). Simultaneous with physical education's achievement of a type of maturity through such legislation, the struggle between the inflexibility of the various foreign systems of gymnastics and the individualistic freedom of the so-called "natural movement" was being waged with increasing vigor. Actually the rising interest in sports and games soon made the conflict unequal, especially when the concept of athletics for all really began to take hold in the second and third decades of the century.

The natural movement was undoubtedly strengthened further by much of the evidence gathered by many natural and social scientists. A certain amount of the spirit of Dewey's philosophy took hold within the educational environment, and this new philosophy and accompanying methodology and techniques did appear to be more effective in the light of the changing ideals of an evolving democracy. Despite this pragmatic influence, however, the influence of idealism remained strong also, with its emphasis on the development of individual personality and the possible inculcation of moral and spiritual values through the transfer of training theory applied to sports and games.

Emergence of the Allied Professions. School health education was developed greatly during the period also. The scope of school hygiene increased, and a required medical examination for all became more important. Leaders were urged to conceive of school health education as including three major divisions: health services, health instruction, and healthful school living. The value of expansion in this area was gradually accepted by educator and citizen alike. For example, many physical educators began to show a concern for a broadening of the field's aims and objectives, the evidence of which could be seen by the increasing amount of time spent by many on coaching duties. Conversely, the expansion of health instruction through the medium of many public and private agencies tended to draw those more directly interested in the goals of health education away from physical education.

Progress in the recreation profession was significant as well. The values inherent in well-conducted playground activities for children and youths were increasingly recognized; the Playground Association of America was organized in 1906. At this time there was still an extremely close relationship between physical education and recreation, a link that remained strong because of the keen interest in the aims of recreation by a number of outstanding physical educators. Many municipal recreation centers were constructed, and it was at this time that the use of some— relatively few, actually—of the schools for "after-hour" recreation began. People began to recognize that recreational activities served an important purpose in a society undergoing basic changes. Some recreation programs developed under local boards of education; others were formed by the joint sponsorship of school boards and municipal governments; and a large number of communities placed recreation under the direct control of the municipal government and either rented school facilities when possible, or gradually developed recreational facilities of their own.

Professional Associations Form Alliance. The American Alliance for Health, Physical Education, Recreation, and Dance) has accomplished a great deal in a strong united effort to coordinate the various allied professions largely within the framework of public and private education. Despite membership losses during the 1970s, the AAHPERD has been a success story promoting those functions which properly belong within the educational sphere. The Alliance should in time through the development of its several national associations also gradually increase its influence on those seeking those services and opportunities that we can provide at the various other age levels as well.

Of course, for better or worse, there are many other health agencies and groups, recreational associations and enterprises, physical education associations and "splinter" disciplinary groups, and athletics associations and organizations moving in a variety of directions. One example of these is the North American Society for Sport Management that began in the mid-1980s that has grown significantly since. Each of these is presumably functioning with the system of values and norms prevailing in the country (or culture, etc.) and the resultant pluralistic educational philosophies extant within such a milieu.

We have also seen teacher education generally, under which physical education has been bracketed, and professional preparation for recreational leadership as well, strengthened through self-evaluation and accreditation. The dance movement has been a significant development within the educational field, and those concerned are still determining the place for this movement within the educational program at all levels. A great deal of progress has been made in physical education, sport, and (more recently) in kinesiology research since 1960.

Achieving Some Historical Perspective

It is now possible to achieve some historical perspective about the second and third quarters of the 20th century as they have affected sport and physical activity education, as well as the allied professions of health education, recreation, and dance education. The Depression of the 1930s, World War II, the Korean War, the Vietnam War, and the subsequent cold war with the many frictions among countries have been strong social forces directly influencing physical education, educational health education, recreation, and dance in any form and in any country to the end of the 20th century. Conversely, to what extent these various fields and their professional concerns have in turn influenced the many cultures, societies, and social systems remains yet to be determined accurately.

It would be simplistic to say (1) that physical activity educators want more and better physical activity education and intramural-recreational sport programs, (2) that athletics-oriented coaches and administrators want more and better athletic competition, (3) that health and safety educators want more and better health and safety education, (4) that recreation personnel want more and better recreation, and (5) that dance educators want more and better dance instruction—and yet, this would probably be a correct assessment of their wishes and probably represents what has occurred to a greater or lesser degree.

As these words are being written, there is still a continuing value struggle going on in the United States that results in characteristic swings of the educational pendulum to and fro. It seems most important that a continuing search for a consensus be carried out. Fortunately, the theoretical struggle fades a bit when actual educational practice is carried out. If this were not so, very little progress would be possible. To continue to strive for improved educational standards for all this should result in the foreseeable future in greater understanding and wisdom on the part of the majority of North American citizens. In this regard science and philosophy can and indeed must make ever-greater contributions.

All concerned members of the so-called *allied* professions in both the United States and Canada (AAHPERD and PHE Canada) need to be fully informed as they strive for a voice in shaping the future development of their respective countries and professions. It is essential that there be careful and continuing study and analysis of the question of values as they relate to sport, exercise, dance, and play. Such study and analysis is, of course, basic as well to the implications that societal values and norms have for the allied fields of health and safety education, recreation, dance, and sport management.

Note: The information about the United States has been adapted from several sources, sections or parts of reports or books written earlier by the author. See Zeigler, 1951, 1962, 1975, 1977, 1979, 1988a, 1988b, 1990, 2003, 2005.

Part VI
The Sport Hero Phenomenon

History has been replete with the exploits of heroes and heroines. It could be argued that a society needs its heroes and heroines as part of its growth and development process, as well as for pattern maintenance. If these leaders don't appear in the normal (abnormal?) course of events (as seems to be the case today), it could be hypothesized further that society will somehow create them in sometimes unexpected places as people fulfill exacting, trying, and unusual roles that are demanded of them.

There appears to be no doubt but that certain, quite specific societal conditions provide greater opportunity for the individual with heroic qualities to emerge (e.g., war, emergencies, crises, competitive sport). Nevertheless, we might agree that such a person might emerge at any time or place if a combination of conditions prevail in any of life's recognized activities.

Please keep in mind that a hero has been defined in the past as "a man [or woman] of distinguished courage or ability admired for his [or her] brave deeds and qualities." A culture hero appears to be a notch higher on the scale, however, and is explained as "a mythicized historical figure who embodies the aspirations or ideals of a society" *(Random House Dictionary*, 1988, p. 488).

In making an attempt to carry out an analysis such as this, the investigator was faced with the fact that several choices would have to be made. For example, it is one thing to describe what a sport hero *was* at some time *in the past*, as opposed to what such a person is *today*. Also, many people would like to see a discussion about what a sport hero(ine) *should be* (in the vain hope that such a wish might actually bring about a change in people's outlooks).

A second choice that was confronted relates to what person or group of persons is making an assessment that so-and-so is indeed a sport hero. A person might believe that Walter Payton of football fame was a sport hero of the finest type in the United States. Citizens of Canada, however, would probably view the great hockey player, Wayne Gretzky, or the late Terry Fox (the one-legged runner suffering from cancer who sought to run across the entire country), eligible for such an honor. Obviously, what country the athlete resides in makes a significant difference! Also, a state or provincial legislature at times passes a resolution about a great athlete, and a university even granted an honorary doctorate to a great hockey goaltender several years ago. Moving to a broader sphere, a belief about a great athlete may be further extended to the national, societal, or world level.

Here, therefore, the author has delimited himself (1) to the delineation of those factors or influences that *should* be considered when (2) a nation gives every indication that it regards a particular man or woman as a sport hero <u>now</u>. (Because it is awkward to continually refer to "sport hero[ine}, hereafter the term "sport hero" will be used, and the reader should understand that both sexes are intended by this term.)

The Hero in Sport

Turning to the topic of the sport hero, consider the situation in the United States in the first half of the twentieth century. If we seek to name a United States sport hero and place him or her in cultural perspective during this time, a great many people would immediately name Babe Ruth as a sport (and culture?) hero in the post-World War I era. In an earlier paper, Zeigler (1987) argued that Lou Gehrig, the Babe's teammate, is actually the person who should have been named as both the sport and the <u>culture</u> hero—and that this recognition should have carried through to the present. Babe Ruth, as the argument goes, should have simply been designated as a great (superb!) athlete. (In 1958, p. 267, Kahn, writing on the topic satirically, stated "Hollywood offers Ava Gardner as Aphrodite; sports gives us Babe Ruth as Zeus.")

Crepeau on Ruth

Eminent sport historian, Dick Crepeau, writing about the "tensions of the twenties", viewed this decade "as an important watershed in the development of the United States." In commenting about George Herman Ruth, Crepeau adds to the image suggested by Kahn above: "Ruth is the essence of the rugged individual playing the national game of the cow pasture in an urban stadium before the cheering masses of the machine age" (Pers. Corres., 2011/01/20).

Building on this statement that seems to epitomize the early 20th-century growth of the world's largest and most powerful capitalistic democracy, it becomes understandable why a number of philosophers and other critics have argued that the United States has had "an idealistic superstructure and a materialistic base!" If this is true, it is probably nowhere more evident than in the way that Babe Ruth and Lou Gehrig, two of the more important "elements" who made up the "Pride of the Yankees," have been evaluated by sport historians and most citizens in the States then and down to the present.

"The Babe" has become a culture hero of the greatest magnitude despite the very obvious, serious flaws in his character, while "Larrupin' Lou," Ruth's teammate, is only remembered fondly by some baseball aficionados as an excellent durable athlete with many fine personality traits. (and also by those who know what amytrophic lateral sclerosis is!)

In assessing the role of sport, however, there have been those who assert that "we have seen the last of the athletic hero" (e.g., London, 1978). Yet, if society "needs heroes," and if they are still emerging in ongoing societal life, is that not reason to believe that a true hero could conceivably emerge in competitive sport? Admittedly, the right (i.e., correct or appropriate) conditions would have to be present (operative in some sequential order?) for the creation (establishment) of such a person. Exactly what might these conditions be?

To obtain some tentative answers from specific scholars, in this paper the disciplines and professions of history, sociology, economics, medicine (psychiatry), anthropology, and philosophy were consulted. (The treatment of sport heroes and heroines in literature could also be analyzed, but that must wait for another time.) Here the investigator received assistance in a form that may help us understand why there seem to be very few heroes in society. Also, it may be discovered why many people are disturbed about what is occurring in sport as one of society's highly visible collectivities. As a part of this discussion, we will be considering such questions as: (a) what factors seem to have an influence in the development of a hero or heroine at any level of society?; (b) do heroes assist in the maintenance of a desirable "moving equilibrium" in Parsons' general action system?; (c) if culture has a need for heroes to assist with "equilibrium maintenance," how can sport heroes serve to fulfill society's need in this respect?; (d) is a sequence or hierarchy of steps required for a person to achieve (i.e. to be declared) a sport hero, and (perhaps) even a folk or culture hero?; and, finally, (e) what might a model look like that could serve as a basis for further investigation?

Insight from History

First, turning to the discipline of history and building on the work of Barney (1984) in which he sought to establish a consensual listing of the "basic tenets" required for the "development" of a hero, the following is a brief summary of what was done. Barney reviewed and analyzed the work of Thomas Carlyle (1840), Friedrich Nietzsche (1958), Dixon Wecter (1941), Sidney Hook (1955), Daniel Boorstin (1961), Orrin Klapp (1972), and Marshall Fishwick (1969, 1975) (not to mention the ancient Greek concept of 'arete'= virtue, meaning excellence not sinlessness). (Nietzsche and Hook will be discussed separately under the heading of "Insight from Philosophy.")

As a result of his investigation, therefore, Barney (1984) concluded that the following was necessary for adjudgement of a man or woman as a contemporary sport hero:

A Bona Fide Sport Hero:

1. Must exemplify *physical excellence* in terms of health, fitness, and skill as an athlete.
2. Must exemplify *moral excellence* in terms of generosity, self-control, and righteousness.
3. Must exhibit *social excellence* in terms of protecting the community before self.
4. Must survive the *judgment* of time with respect to *all* of the above.

Thomas Carlyle (n.d.), a Scotsman who is still recognized for his interest in the role of great men in the shaping of history, has provided us with the classic description of the hero in a series of lectures given in 1840. For him, the hero was a man who took control of an evolving situation. He described their manner of appearance in our world's business, how they have shaped themselves in the world's history, what ideas men formed of them, what work they did… they are the leaders of men, these great ones; the modelers, patterns, and in a wide sense creators, of whatsoever the general mass of men contrived to do or attain… the soul of the whole world's history… (pp. 1-2)).

Insight from Sociology

Turning to the discipline of *sociology*, Johnson (1969) discussed the great importance of values and norms in a society. He explained that there were four subsystems within the total action system defined by Parsons and others (i.e., cultural system, social system, psychological system, and behavioral-organic system). Moreover, there are also <u>four</u> levels within that subsystem that has been identified as the social system or structure. These levels, proceeding from "highest" to "lowest," are (a) values, (b) norms, (c) the structure of collectivities, and (d) the structure of roles. Typically the higher levels are more general than the lower ones, with the latter group giving quite specific guidance to those segments or units of the particular system to which they apply. These "units" or "segments" are either collectivities or individuals in their capacity as role occupants (e.g., the hero and—conceivably—the sports hero).

Values are, therefore, extremely important and represent the highest echelon of the social system level of the entire general action system. These values may be categorized into such "entities" as artistic values, educational values, social values (including sport values), etc. Of course, all types or categories of values must be values <u>of</u> personalities. The social values of a particular social system are those values that are conceived of as representative of the ideal general character that is desired by those who ultimately hold the power in the system being described. The most important social values in North America, for example, have been (1) the rule of law, (2) the socio-structural facilitation of individual achievement, and (3) the equality of opportunity (Johnson, 48).

Functional Interchanges. A society is the most nearly self-subsistent type of social system and, interestingly enough again, societies or "live systems or personalities" typically have four basic types of functional problems involving functional interchange (each with its appropriate value principle). The one that concerns us directly here is the pattern-maintenance problem that has to do with the inculcation of the value system and the maintenance of the social system's commitment to it (Parsons, *et al.*, 1961, pp. 38-41. Presumably, society uses its heroes to help in pattern-maintenance. And, if they aren't readily available—as seems to be the case at present—it creates them in various ways. Generally, therefore, these interchange processes are the means by which a society's production factors are related, combined, and transformed with *utility*—the value principle of the adaptive system—as the interim product. These products "packaged" as various forms of "utility" are employed in and by other functional subsystems of the society.

In describing how each process is carried out in a social system, Zetterberg (1968) likens any such assessment to the examination of four master gauges controlling the social system. If the dial on any one gauge didn't maintain a minimum value and fell into a "danger zone," the whole system would fail. Conversely, when all dials are operating "safely," any significant advancement in one problem area would need to be matched by the others. In this way a "moving equilibrium" would be maintained.

Thus, if we were to carry such theorizing further, the possible contribution of sociological theory in this vein in regard to the role of the heroic person would be as follows: a hero's contribution to society would be in the nature of serving (disproportionately?) to help society to maintain a "moving equilibrium" among the various subsystems controlling the social system.

Insight from Economics

Moving from the consideration of the ideal role for a hero to fulfill, Veblen (1899), writing satirically as an economics and business theorist with heavy sociological and psychological overtones, argued that, conversely, the sports hero can emerge from activities provided within a culture for developmental purposes:

> . . . those members of respectable society who advocate
> athletic games commonly justify their attitude on this
> head to themselves and to their neighbors on the
> ground that these games serve as an invaluable means
> of development. They not only improve the
> contestant's physique, but it is commonly added that
> they also foster a manly spirit, both in the participants
> and the spectators. . .

Although he sees the budding athlete as "emotionally immature," nevertheless,

> The physical vigor acquired in the training for athletic games—so far
> as the training may be said to have this effect— is of advantage to both

116

the individual and the collectivity, in that, other things being equal, it conduces to serviceability. The spiritual traits which go with athletic sports are likewise economically advantageous to the individual as contradistinguished from the interests of the collectivity ...

Accordingly, Veblen finds that:

> Modern competition is in large a process of self-assertion on the basis of these traits of predatory human nature. In the sophisticated form in which they enter into the modern, peaceable emulation, the possession of these traits in some measure is almost a necessary of life to the civilized man... (pp. 173-175).

In assessing situation in the late 20th century, however, Cuff (1983) argued that the role of the *professional* athlete has not changed significantly since Veblen expressed his opinion about (largely) college and semiprofessional sport. "There are more of them," he states, "earning more money and performing for more people, but the image and the marketing of the sport is still pre-eminent, more important than the game itself" (p, 3).

Insight from Anthropology

Henry (1963), writing from an anthropological perspective, explained that "The central activity of all cultures is always a self-maximizing machine ("ego-building"), whether it be the ceremonial exchange of necklaces and arm bands as in the famous kula of the Trobriand Islands in the South Pacific, the economic competition of business in our culture, or the rat-race to get one's articles and books published in the American academic world" (p. 191). Building on this theory, Henry explained that athletics achieves status in that the outstanding athletes on the teams generate varying quantities of "self-substance" for whomever they represent at whichever level of society. Interestingly, also, the fan is "enhanced" when the team wins, is disappointed when the team loses, but "its failure does not touch him at his core" (p. 191). In summary, sport is (can be) an important part of a community's, school's, university's, state's, or nation's self-maximizing system.

Insight from Psychiatry

In Freud's work there are themes of heroism and weakness. For him the hero has few doubts internally; life's conflicts are out there in the external world, and he meets them head-on. In his sexual relationships, an aspect of life so basic in Freud's thought, this person has a vast amount of energy potential and finds ready release for unconscious desire and conscious satisfaction of instinctual needs. In Riesman's analysis (1954) of this subject, "the ego of the hero is in unquestioned demand, and that conflict between the conscious and the unconscious levels of the personality is at a minimum" (p. 252). This Freudian hero could well be found playing an important role in a Spartan-like manner in an Ayn Rand novel such as *The Fountainhead*. He is oriented toward reality, and he is a "winner." The world is very much aware that this individual has been part of it and its development.

Insight from Philosophy

Shifting attention to the discipline of philosophy for possible further enlightenment, Nietzsche, the nineteenth century philosopher, appeared to view the hero as a great cultural figure in similar fashion to the position taken by Carlyle (see above). According to such theory, Providence seems to have provided for humankind at appropriate points in history. Such a great man (person) was a "world-historical" person (Hegel) through whom Reason (according to this world view) operated. This person helped to shape history for the betterment of humankind by his actions, thereby providing a noble ideal for all people to follow. Nietzsche's Superman was "a notch above" his fellows; "what he tried above all to promote was the supremacy of the man who was best, that is healthiest and strongest in character" (Russell, 1959, p. 258).

A mid-20th-century philosopher, Sidney Hook, has made a significant contribution to the role played by the hero in history (1955). Hook's hero is a person who has heroic qualities and then sets out deliberately to influence the course of human events in a particular sphere of action. This person is more than "Johnny on the spot" when a brave act is needed; he or she consciously brings heroic qualities to bear in order to alter the course of events in some phase of life. Status as a hero is earned within a larger social context (p. 154).

Tiger Woods Was Caught in a Vise

A word of caution is needed here, however, because of the obvious complexity of the decision-making process is arriving at an objective conclusion in this matter. A value criterion for greatness or "heroic stature" may be most difficult to establish. Nevertheless, because of its importance in society, we should be able to work toward different, but appropriate, definitions of a hero functioning in different spheres of social life.

A perfect example that demonstrates the extreme complexity of the subject at hand arose very recently in the case of the world's top golfer, Tiger Woods.

The Occurrence. Tiger Woods, a young man in his thirties, had become a household name because of his great success as a professional golfer. He was named the outstanding golf professional of the 2000-2009 decade and undoubtedly was a "golden boy" in the sporting world. However, he had been leading a double life. Presumably happily married to a beautiful Swedish wife with two lovely children, and on the way to becoming fabulously wealthy, Woods had an automobile accident outside of his home in the early hours of a morning. This mishap subsequently brought to light a tale of extraordinary, "extracurricular" sexual activity with many mistresses far and wide.

This scandal immediately became one of the top media stories of the year 2009. The public was surprised and also startled. In fairly short order, the "miscreant" felt constrained to offer a public apology and to take an indefinite leave from his work as professional gold player. The implications resulting from this move away from the "world of golf" were potentially devastating to both the future of Woods himself and to the development of the sport of golf.

Why Was This Story So Newsworthy? Watching this scandal mature over several months, I asked myself: "Why is this such a 'big deal'?" Is this development so unusual in the history of the world? Haven't various media personalities, including sport figures, experienced problems of this type before? Why is this particular incident worthy of all this attention? (Note: The ethical aspect of his relationship with Dr. Galea in Toronto who administered PEDs in Toronto to speed up Tiger's recovery from knee surgery is not considered here.) The answer is that this incident is not *unique*, but it is *unusual.*

Yet, one wonders why has so much public attention been given to this particular situation? I believe the answer can be found in the fact that, in the past one hundred years, the role of sport in society has changed so radically. Competitive sport and related physical activity has gradually, but steadily, become a *social institution* that surged enormously in importance. Sport has become an extremely powerful social force that must be reckoned with from here into the indeterminate future.

Because of this upsurge in sport's development, I have personally been attempting to analyze it from a socio-cultural perspective. It appears to be a question of the "use of" and the "abuse of" of sport. The underlying theoretical argument that can be made is as follows: Strong institutions (i.e., "forces" or "influences") govern society. Among those social institutions are:

(1) society's values (including created norms
     based on these values),
(2) the type of political state in vogue,
(3) the prevailing economic system,
(4) the religious beliefs present, etc.

To these longstanding institutions, I have over the years added such other influences as education, the communication media, science and technological advancement, concern for peace, *and now sport itself.* Of all of these, the values a society holds, and the accompanying norms developed on the basis of these values, form the strongest institution of all!

Hard Questions About Present Social Institutions. Social institutions are created and nurtured within a society ostensibly to further the positive development of the people living within that culture. Take democracy, for example, as a type of political institution that is currently being promoted vigorously by the United States throughout the entire world. (Of course, such worldwide change will take time!) Within this form of social development, democracy has also developed a strong relationship with economics– especially with the institution of capitalism. Economics, of course, is another vital social institution upon which a society depends fundamentally.

As world civilization developed, a great many of the world's countries have enacted with almost messianic zeal the promotion of such social institutions as democracy, capitalism, and—now—an increasing involvement with the promotion of competitive sport. The "theory" behind such promotion is that the addition of highly competitive sport to this mix will bring about more "good" than "bad" for the people and the countries involved. However, this social experiment has raised a number of disturbing questions that society must consider.

Underlying the rampant promotion of commercialized sport, of course, is this possibly questionable alliance of democracy and rampant capitalism. Think of the example being set in North America, for example. Is there reasonable hope that this present brand of "democratic capitalism" that uses up the world's environmental resources inordinately will somehow improve the world situation in the long run? Can we truly claim with any degree of certainty that this "mix" of democracy and capitalism (with its subsequent inclusion of big-time sport) is producing more "good" than "bad"? (Admittedly, we do need to delineate between "what's 'good'" and "what's 'bad'" more carefully). There is no escaping the fact that the gap economically between the rich and the poor is steadily increasing. This means that "the American dream for all"–what was known as "the Enlightenment Ideal"–is beginning to look like a desert mirage for the "good, old USA".

What Happened to the "Enlightenment Ideal"? Recall that the late 18th century was a time of political revolution when monarchies, aristocracies, and the ecclesiastical structure were being challenged on a number of fronts. In addition, the factory system was undergoing significant change at that time. Such industrial development with its greatly improved machinery "coincided with the formulation and diffusion of the modern Enlightenment idea of history as a record of progress. …" Hence, this "new scientific knowledge and technological power was expected to make possible a comprehensive improvement in all of the conditions of life—social, political, moral, and intellectual as well as material" ([Leo] Marx).

This idea did slowly take hold and eventually "became the fulcrum of the dominant American worldview" (p. 5). By 1850, however, with the rapid growth of the United States especially, *the idea of progress was already being dissociated from the Enlightenment vision of political and social liberation.*
Then, by the turn of the century (1900), "the technocratic idea of progress [had become] a belief in the sufficiency of scientific and technological innovation as the basis for general progress." This came to mean that if scientific-based technologies were permitted to develop in an unconstrained manner, there would be an automatic improvement in all other aspects of life!

What had happened—because this theory became coupled with onrushing, unbridled capitalism—was that the ideal envisioned by Thomas Jefferson *had been turned upside down*! Instead of social progress being guided by *such values as justice, freedom, and self-fulfillment for all*, these goals of vital interest in a democracy were subjugated to a burgeoning society dominated by supposedly more important *instrumental* values.

As it developed, America's chief criterion of progress has undergone a subtle but decisive change since the founding of the Republic. That change is at once a cause and a reflection of much of the current disenchantment by many with advancement in technology. Hence, the fundamental question today could well be: "Which values will win out in the long run?" Will the historical "Enlightenment Ideal" remain as an unfulfilled dream forever?

Challenging the Role of Sport in Society. Now, returning to "the Tiger Woods Saga", we find Tiger as a prominent figure in sport, a social institution whose influence has increased phenomenally. This development has become so vast that we may now ask whether it is accomplishing what it is presumably supposed to do. Is highly competitive sport as a social phenomenon doing more good than harm in society? The world seems to have accepted as fact that it is! Yet the world community does not really know whether this contention is true or not. Sport's expansion is permitted and encouraged almost without question in all quarters. "Sport is good for people, and more involvement with sport of almost any type—extreme sport, professional wrestling, missed martial arts, 'world cups'—is better" seems to be the conventional wisdom. Witness, in addition, the billions of dollars that are being removed neatly out of tax revenues for the several Olympic enterprises perennially.

As I analyzed the "Tiger Woods Saga," I found it impossible to avoid a critique of commercialized sport as well. I believe that the development is now such that society should be striving to keep sport's drawbacks and/or excesses in check to the greatest possible extent. In recent decades we have witnessed the rise of sport throughout the land to the status of a fundamentalist religion. For example, we find sport being called upon to serve as a "redeemer of wayward youth," but—as it is occurring elsewhere—I believe it is also becoming a destroyer of certain fundamental values of individual and social life.

Wilcox, for example, in his empirical analysis, challenged "the widely held notion that sport can fulfill an important role in the development of national character." He stated: "the assumption that sport is conducive to the development of positive human values, or the 'building of character,' should be viewed more as a belief rather than as a fact." He concluded that sport did "provide some evidence to support a relationship between participation in sport and the ranking of human values" (1991, pp. 3, 17, 18, respectively).

Assuming Wilcox's view has reasonable validity, those involved in any way in the institution of sport—if they all together may be considered a collectivity—should contribute a quantity of redeeming social value to our North American culture, not to mention the overall world culture (i.e., a quantity of good leading to improved societal well-being). On the basis of this argument, the following two questions can be postulated for response by concerned agencies and individuals (e.g., federal governments, state and provincial officials, philosophers in the discipline and related professions):

(1) Can, does, or should a great (i.e., leading) nation produce great sport?

(2) With the world being threatened environmentally in a variety of ways, should we now be considering the "ecology" of sport as we are doing with other human activity? Both the beneficial and disadvantageous aspects of a particular sporting activity should be studied through the endeavors of scholars in various disciplines as well?

(3) If it is indeed the case that the guardian of the "functional satisfaction" resulting from sport is (a) the sports person, (b) the spectator, (c) the businessperson who gains monetarily, (d) the sport manager, and, in some instances, (e) educational administrators and their respective governing boards, then who in society should be in a position to be the most knowledgeable about the immediate objectives and long range aims of sport and related physical activity?

Answering these questions is a complex matter. First, as stated above, sport and related physical activity have become an extremely powerful social force in society. Secondly, if we grant that sport now has significant power in all world cultures—a power indeed that appears to be growing—we should also recognize that any such social force affecting society is dangerous if perverted (e.g., through an excess of nationalism or commercialism). With this in mind, I am arguing further that sport has somehow achieved such status as a powerful societal institution without an adequately defined underlying theory. Somehow, most countries seem to be proceeding generally on a typically unstated assumption that "sport is a good thing for society to encourage, and *more* sport is even better!" And yet, as explained above, the term "sport" exhibits radical ambiguity based on both everyday usage and dictionary definition. This obviously adds even more to the present problem and accompanying confusion.

This "radical ambiguity" about the role of sport takes us back to "the Tiger Woods Saga". Sport has now become a powerful social institution exerting influence for the betterment of society. Then, all of a sudden, a "sport hero" of the highest magnitude behaves himself in such a way that basic societal values are challenged. Hence, we now must ask ourselves: "Specifically what are *the* values that Tiger has forsaken that have occasioned this world-wide outburst of publicity"?

"Socio-Instrumental", Material Values or "Moral", Non-Material Values? Examining this matter carefully, we may be surprised to learn that sport's contribution to human wellbeing is a highly complicated matter. On the one side, there are those who claim that sport contributes significantly to the development of what are regarded as the *socio-economic, material values*—that is, the values of teamwork, loyalty, self-sacrifice, aggressiveness, and perseverance consonant with prevailing corporate capitalism in democracy and in other political systems as well. In the process of making this "contribution," however, we discover also that there is now a good deal of evidence that in the process of contributing to the "global ideal" of capitalism, democracy, and advancing technology, sport has developed an ideal that opposes the historical, fundamental ***moral***, *non-material values* of honesty, fairness, good will, sportsmanship, and responsibility in the innumerable competitive experiences provided (Lumpkin, Stoll, and Beller, 1999).

Significant to this discussion are the results of investigations carried out by Hahm, Stoll, Beller, Rudd, and others in recent years. The Hahm-Beller Choice Inventory (HBVCI) has now been administered to athletes at different levels in a variety of venues. It demonstrates conclusively that athletes are increasingly ***not*** supporting what is considered "the moral ideal" in competition. As Stoll and Beller (1998) reported, for example, an athlete with moral character demonstrates the moral character traits of honesty, fair play, respect, and responsibility whether an official is present to enforce the rules or not. (Priest, Krause, and Beach substantiated this finding in 1999). They reported that changes over a four-year period in a college athlete's ethical value choices were consistent with other investigations. Their findings showed *decreases* in "sportsmanship orientation" and an *increase* in "professional" attitudes associated with sport bespeaking so-called "social" values..

Aha! We have now arrived at the nub of the matter! Alas for poor Tiger Woods… His plight is that he is "caught" right in the middle of this ongoing controversy about the presumed contribution of sport. No matter which way he turns, he is "out of step" with the claims for sport made by either group. His actions clash with those who say that sport contributes to **socio-economic**, *material* values.

> Note: Please note that I am recommending a change in the terminology used. The distinction made between the two types of values has been most insightful. However, I believe that the term "socio-economic"–rather than simply "socio-instrumental" (or even "material!) would more accurately reflect what has taken place in society

The perennial winner in golf, poor Tiger can't win now for losing! On the one hand he has confounded those who argue for "the socio-instrumental-values contribution", and–on the other hand–he has betrayed those who promote sport because it makes "a moral-values contribution". Hence, advertisers are now deserting Tiger "in droves" because his commercial value to them has been tarnished irrevocably. The gross stock value of his many sponsors has decreased appreciably since Tiger has been exposed. Concurrently, the sports *hero*, that staunch fellow presumably with all of those fine moral values, has betrayed his fans young and old because of his presumed "nocturnal peregrinations." Woe is Tiger!

Proposed Tables and Model to Ascertain the Status of Sport Hero

Finally, based on the admittedly, not fully comprehensive material gleaned from this amalgam of scholarly inputs, along with the consideration of the complex Tiger Woods case, the following preliminary model was devised to describe this social phenomenon based on possible knowledge and wisdom gleaned from the representative of these scholarly fields. This proposed model is quite different from the "hypothetical model" or consensual listing proposed by Barney of qualities and/or characteristics required for "judging contemporary candidates for sport heroism" correctly or adequately. A logical—even though embryonic—model is designed as an empirical system to the greatest possible extent. Accordingly it must have boundaries corresponding to the social system being described. This means that boundary-determining criteria are required initially so that the same initial conditions can (presumably) be correlated finally. These criteria are succinctly indicated below based on the above explanation as (1) 19th & 20th Centuries Analyses of Necessary Qualities for Sport Hero Designation, (2) Society's Values & Norms, (3) Personal Situation (Internal Pressures), and (4) Social Situation (External Pressures) (see Tables 1, 2, 3, & 4 below).

TABLE 1
PAST EXPERIENCE: 19TH & 20TH CENTURIES
ANALYSES OF NECESSARY QUALITIES FOR
SPORT HERO(DESIGNATION
(RECOMMENDED
by R.K. BARNEY)

1. MUST EXEMPLIFY <u>PHYSICAL EXCELLENCE</u> IN TERMS OF HEALTH, FITNESS, AND SKILL AS AN ATHLETE.

2. MUST EXEMPLIFY <u>MORAL EXCELLENCE</u> IN TERMS OF GENEROSITY, SELF-CONTROL, AND RIGHTEOUSNESS.

3. MUST EXHIBIT <u>SOCIAL EXCELLENCE</u> IN TERMS OF PROTECTING THE INTERESTS OF THE COMMUNITY BEFORE SELF.

4. MUST SURVIVE THE JUDGEMENT OF TIME WITH RESPECT TO <u>ALL</u> OF THE ABOVE.

TABLE 2

SOCIETY'S (THE UNITED STATES')
VALUE AND NORMS (AS DESIGNATED
from
HARRY M. JOHNSON)

VALUES - THIS IS THE HIGHEST LEVEL OF THE SOCIAL SYSTEM LEVEL OF
THE ENTIRE GENERAL ACTION SYSTEM. PARSONS CATEGORIZES
VALUES (E.G., SCIENTIFIC VALUES, ARTISTIC VALUES, [SPORT VALUES?],
AND VALUES FOR PERSONALITIES).

SOCIAL VALUES ARE CONCEPTIONS OF THE IDEAL GENERAL
CHARACTER OF THE TYPE OF SOCIAL SYSTEM IN QUESTION. FOR THE
U.S., IMPORTANT SOCIETAL VALUES ARE:

(1) THE RULE OF LAW
(2) THE SOCIAL STRUCTURAL FACILITATION
OF INDIVIDUAL ACHIEVEMENT
(3) THE EQUALITY OF OPPORTUNITY

NORMS - SHARED SANCTIONED NORMS ARE THE SECOND LEVEL OF
SOCIAL STRUCTURE. IN THE U.S., EXAMPLES OF NORMS ARE:

(1) THE INSTITUTIONS OF PRIVATE
PROPERTY
(2) PRIVATE ENTERPRISE
(3) THE MONOGAMOUS CONJUGAL FAMILY
(4) THE SEPARATION OF CHURCH AND STATE

TABLE 3
PERSONAL SITUATION (INTERNAL PRESSURES)

"OPINIONS, ATTITUDES, AND BELIEFS ARE MORE
DIFFERENTIATED IN MORE COMPLEX SOCIETIES"
(BERELSON & STEINER, 1964, P. 559) (REPEATED
IN BOTH TABLES 3 AND 4).

"THERE ARE DIFFERENCES IN OPINIONS, ATTITUDES
AND BELIEFS THAT DERIVE FROM THE SOCIAL STRATA
IN WHICH PEOPLE FIND THEMSELVES OR FROM THE
SOCIAL CHARACTERISTICS THAT THEY HAVE" (P. 570).

"PEOPLE HOLD OPINIONS, ATTITUDES, AND BELIEFS
IN HARMONY WITH THEIR GROUP MEMBERSHIP AND
IDENTIFICATION" (BERELSON & STEINER, 1964, P. 566).

"OPINIONS, ATTITUDES, AND BELIEFS ARE 'INHERITED'
FROM ONE'S PARENTS: PEOPLE LEARN THEM EARLY AND
THE LEARNING PERSISTS INTO ADULTHOOD" (P. 562).

"OAB'S WITHIN A GROUP ARE PARTICULARLY SUBJECT TO
INFLUENCE BY THE MOST RESPECTED AND PRESTIGIOUS
MEMBER OF THE GROUP, THE OPINION LEADERS"(P. 569).

"PEOPLE TEND TO MISPERCEIVE AND MISINTERPRET
PERSUASIVE COMMUNICATION IN ACCORDANCE WITH
THEIR OWN PREDISPOSITIONS, BY EVADING THE MESSAGE
OR BY DISTORTING IT IN A FAVORABLE DIRECTION" (P. 536).

OAB'S, AND ESPECIALLY BELIEFS, CHANGE MORE SLOWLY
THAN ACTUAL BEHAVIOR" (P. 576).

"THE MORE INTERESTED PEOPLE ARE IN AN ISSUE, THE
MORE LIKELY THEY ARE TO HOLD CONSISTENT POSITIONS
ON THAT ISSUE" (P. 574).

"AS A CHILD GROWS UP, HE GROWS AWAY FROM THE
ORIGINAL PARENTAL INFLUENCE TO THE EXTENT THAT
HE COMES INTO CONTACT WITH NEW WAYS OF LIFE, NEW
SOCIAL GROUPS, NEW COMMUNITY ENVIRONMENTS,
ETC." (P. 564).

"WHEN PEOPLE'S OAB'S DO NOT HANG TOGETHER
HARMONIOUSLY, THEY ARE MORE LIKELY TO CHANGE
SOME OF THEM" (P. 578).

NOTE: BECAUSE OF THE DIFFICULTY OF DETERMINING WHERE
INDIVIDUAL PSYCHOLOGY "LEAVES OFF" AND SOCIAL
PSYCHOLOGY "BEGIN," SEVERAL FINDINGS ABOUT HUMAN
BEHAVIOR ARE REPEATED IN BOTH TABLE 3 AND TABLE 4.

TABLE 4
SOCIAL SITUATION (EXTERNAL PRESSURES)

"OPINIONS, ATTITUDES, AND BELIEFS ARE MORE
DIFFERENTIATED IN MORE COMPLEX SOCIETIES"
(BERELSON & STEINER, 1964, P. 559).

"GIVEN CONSISTENT SUPPORT FROM HISTORICAL,
PARENTAL, GROUP AND STRATA CHARACTERISTICS,
OAB'S ARE UNLIKELY TO CHANGE AT ALL" (P.575).

"FOR A POPULATION AS A WHOLE, THERE APPEARS
TO BE LITTLE LASTING DEVELOPMENT OF OPINIONS,
ATTITUDES AND BELIEFS THAT IS INDEPENDENT OF
PARENTAL, GROUP, OR STRATA PREDISPOSITIONS
AND IS BASED MAINLY ON 'OBJECTIVE' OR 'RATIONAL'
ANALYSIS OF INFORMATION AND IDEAS" (P. 574).

"PEOPLE HOLD OAB'S IN HARMONY WITH THEIR
GROUP MEMBERSHIPS AND IDENTIFICATIONS" (P. 566).

"THE USE, AND PERHAPS THE EFFECTIVENESS, OF
DIFFERENT MEDIA VARIES WITH THE EDUCATIONAL
LEVEL OF THE AUDIENCE—THE HIGHER THE EDUCATION,
THE GREATER THE RELIANCE ON PRINT; THE LOWER THE
EDUCATION, THE GREATER THE RELIANCE ON AURAL AND
PICTURE MEDIA. THE BETTER EDUCATED ARE MORE
LIKELYTHAN OTHERS TO PAY ATTENTION TO SERIOUS
COMMUNICATIONS DEALING WITH AESTHETIC OR MORAL
OR EDUCATIONAL ISSUES" (P. 533).

"THE MASS MEDIA EXERCISE AN IMPORTANT INDIRECT
INFLUENCE THROUGH 'OPINION LEADERS'-THOSE
TRUSTED AND INFORMED PEOPLE WHO EXIST IN
VIRTUALLY ALL PRIMARY GROUPS" (P. 550).

"THE HIGHER A PERSON'S LEVEL OF INTELLIGENCE,
THE MORE LIKELY IT IS THAT HE WILL ACQUIRE
INFORMATION FROM COMMUNICATION" (P. 544).

"THE MORE TRUSTWORTHY, CREDIBLE, OR PRES-
TIGIOUS THE COMMUNICATOR IS PERCEIVED TO
BE, THE LESS MANIPULATIVE HIS INTENT IS CON-
SIDERED TO BE AND THE GREATER THE IMMEDIATE
TENDENCY TO ACCEPT HIS CONCLUSIONS" (P. 537).

"THE ATTRIBUTION OF A POSITION TO 'MAJORITY
OPINION' IS ITSELF EFFECTIVE IN CHANGING
ATTITUDES WHEN THE AUDIENCE RESPECTS THE GROUP
FROM WHICH THE MAJORITY IS TAKEN" (P. 538).

"AS FOR POLITICAL AFFAIRS, WHAT IS TYPICALLY LEARNED
OR PASSED ON, FROM FATHER (USUALLY) TO CHILD, IS NOT
SO MUCH IDEOLOGY AS A PARTY AFFILIATION" (P. 564).

"OAB'S ARE MORE SUBJECT TO CHANGE WHEN PEOPLE
ARE SUBJECT TO CROSS-PRESSURES" (P. 580).

"PEOPLE RESPOND TO PERSUASIVE COMMUNICATION
IN LINE WITH THEIR PRESENT PREDISPOSITION, AND
THEY CHANGE OR RESIST CHANGE ACCORDINGLY" (P. 540)

In Figure 1 (see below), the common syllogism was used as an illustration of units that share the same boundary-determining criteria (Dubin, 1978, pp. 125-142). Thus: "All people have opinions, attitudes, and beliefs [they think!]; a potential sport hero (ine) is one person functioning within the total population; therefore, people are in a position to form opinions, attitudes, and beliefs about the qualities of such a person." Also, those historical, social, and individual factors were employed with appropriate headings (as explained in Tables 1-4 inclusive) as they appear to influence a person's eventual designation as hero(ine) by the society in which he or she lives.

One of the first things that became clear was the extreme complexity of such a designation in an open society (e.g., the United States, Canada, certain European countries). North American culture, for example, is characterized by pluralistic philosophies with departmental philosophies subsumed under each recognizable philosophic position. Obviously, the impact of the various components (e.g., society's values and norms) of the model would be quite different in a managed society characterized by a more authoritarian form of government. When a democratic society decides that so-and-so is a sport hero, this is the result of a great many factors, influences, and relationships that at certain points become an intricate network. Thus, arriving at the final designation by society is a highly complex matter and is obviously the result of a great many determinants of greater or lesser importance. To grasp one or two such factors and state that "it was either this or that which brought about John Jones' or Mary Smith's designation as a sport hero in the community of Plainville, Nebraska is to truly misunderstand the problem." Some time in the future, someone may attempt to determine the relative weighting of the various determinants by factor analysis—but even then the reader probably shouldn't bet on the infallible accuracy of such a determination.

FIGURE 1

FACTORS INFLUENCING SPORT HERO DESIGNATION IN TODAY'S WORLD

SOCIETY'S PRESENT
VALUES & NORMS

19TH & 20TH
HISTORICAL
ANALYSES

INFLUENCE OF

PERSONAL
SITUATION_____EXTERNAL
(INTERNAL   SITUATION
PRESSURES)   (SOCIAL
                                                  PRESSURES)

DESIGNATION AS A SPORT HERO!

Even though dictionaries define *social* character similarly, sport practitioners, including participants, coaches, parents, and officials, have gradually come to believe that character is defined properly by such values as self-sacrifice, teamwork, loyalty, and perseverance. The common expression in competitive sport is: "He or she showed character"—meaning "He/she 'hung in there' to the bitter end!" [or whatever…]. Rudd et al. (1999) confirmed that coaches explained character as "work ethic and commitment." This coincides with what sport sociologists have found. Sage (1998. p. 614) explained: "Mottoes and slogans such as 'sports builds character' must be seen in the light of their ideological issues." In other words, competitive sport is structured by the nature of the society in which it occurs. This would appear to mean that over-commercialization, drug-taking, cheating, bribe-taking by officials, violence, etc. at all levels of sport are simply reflections of the culture in which we live.

Where does all of this leave us today as we consider sport's presumed relationship with *moral* character development and with *social* character development? Whatever your conclusion may be, Tiger Woods has been unexpectedly trapped in this social-moral character vise that characterizes sport participation at the beginning of the 21st century. He tried to have it both ways. For his and his family's sake, let us hope that he will learn from this tragic experience—and that "the world" will "forgive his sins"…

Concluding Statement

Times are indeed changing. Whereas at various times throughout history, the world had its Hercules, Samson, Beowulf, and Siegfried, Stark (1987) concluded that, in Western culture, Stallone (whether Rocky or Rambo) served to reinforce our conception of the heroes who emerged in recent years. "Many scholars, for example, place Mr. Stallone squarely in the footsteps of John Wayne, Clint Eastwood, and Arnold Schwarzenegger, and say his heroes display much of the same rugged, macho individualism as the old heroes of westerns . . ." (p, 19). These are examples of how one individual reacted to a world where society has lost control and thereby has failed its citizens.

Frankly, this topic of sport hero was examined because it does seem that this question is unclear in the minds of most citizens, young or old, including the athletes themselves. People need to understand through use of their own rational powers that they are being increasingly lured or marketed daily by others into reactions dominated more by emotions than reason. It may well be necessary to reinforce ego at the various geographical levels (i.e. community, region, state or province, nation) by the creation of heroes in the various aspects of social living (including sport). To what extent this should be done through the artificial creation of Superman, WonderWoman, Rambo, Spiderman, and Indiana Jones is debatable. In addition, as it developed, even Tiger Woods defaulted after having achieved "superstar" but not hero status. However, it may serve a beneficial purpose when such individuals do not appear normally in the course of ongoing events.

Further, if this is what is happening in competitive sport, we might ask to what extent highly competitive sport is indeed a "socially useful servant" today? We know how difficult it is to make a case for the building of desirable character and personality traits through the medium of sport. Our values often seem to have become so perverted that we *condone* certain unsportsmanlike and illegal actions in sport and athletics at any level, and then turn right around and condemn, fine, and even send to jail people who display similar behavior in everyday life? Permitting unethical and illegal behavior in sport is a serious mistake. Intelligent, influential people must become very concerned about this anomaly in social life. Competitive sport has become an increasingly important social force in the world—almost too great an influence if this is possible. Further, culture heroes are truly hard to come by these days. If we really believe that sport has an important contribution to make to the development of a fine society, is it not time to give the highest reward and acclaim to whose who demonstrate through sport *both* a high degree of athletic ability <u>and</u> the finest of personality and character traits. We should give high priority to bringing about a change in the present state of affairs as soon as possible

Scott Silvers, of Kansas City, Missouri, in a letter to *Sports Illustrated* in the late 20th century (Oct. 29, 1984) about Walter Payton's (a Chicago Bear) new rushing record in professional football, stated: "I'm sure that many of your readers will be nominating him for Sportsman of the Year. Nobody deserves it more… The term 'sportsman' implies traits that go beyond athleticism: humility, kindness, generosity. A true sportsman is someone who combines these personal attributes with athletic ability . . ." (p. 110). Adding a "hero connotation" to this to me implies the addition of extraordinary courage or ability, admired for "brave deeds and noble qualities." If sport participants such as this were given the type of recognition they deserve, we would be in a much better position to argue logically that highly competitive sport is indeed an important useful social force. However, if we continue to condone (as we often look the other way) distasteful, unsportsmanlike, overly mercenary actions in sport, we are simply affirming the negative aspects of sport as an entertainment device in an otherwise (presumably) boring existence.

Finally, it may well be an important responsibility of sport historians to help people separate the true heroes and heroines from the celebrities. We have a condition prevailing in which the media offer us the "packaged hero" for consumption. We were told in 1975 by Fishwick that the hero is a reflection of the place and the era in which he lives. Thus, despite the fact that the media needs celebrity figures to sell their wares, and despite the fact that politicians need a variety of symbols that are somehow supposed to reflect glory on them, the people themselves must insist that heroes and heroines, in sport or any other aspect of life, truly reflect the finest societal values that we proclaim for our culture. As London (1978) stated, "The hero is an extinct species relegated to the memory of my youthful idealism… This is the age of the superstar, not the hero. And superstars specialize in self-adulation, not sacrifice." In one of her well-known songs, songstress Peggy Lee said it all with one plaintive question—"Is that all there is?"

Part VII
The Olympic Games:
A Question of Values

There's a vocal minority who believe the Olympic Games should be abolished. There's another minority, including the Games officials and the athletes, who obviously feel the enterprise is doing just fine. In addition, there's a larger minority undoubtedly solidly behind the commercial aspects of the undertaking. They have a good thing going; they liked the Games the way they are developing—the bigger, the better! Finally, there's the vast majority to whom the Olympics are either interesting, somewhat interesting, or a bore. This "vast majority," if the Games weren't "there!" every four years, would probably agree that the world would go on just the same, and some other social phenomenon would take up their leisure time.

Ancient Olympism

Olympism has its roots in the beliefs of the ancient Greeks, who encouraged people to develop their physical, moral, intellectual, cultural and artistic qualities harmoniously. This meant taking part in a blend of sport, art, educational and cultural activities. This philosophy was celebrated through the Olympic Games, a festival involving athletes, scholars and artists from many cultural fields.

The (Intended) Goal of Modern Olympism

Frenchman Pierre de Coubertin, who in 1894 led the re-establishment of the Olympic Movement, is recognized as the father of modern Olympism. He modernized ancient Greek ideals and launched them again to the rest of the world through the staging of a modern Olympic Games in 1896. Today, the festival celebrates the ideals that remain at the heart of Olympism. By blending sport with culture and education, Olympism promotes a way of life based on:

> The balanced development of the body, will and mind
> The joy found in effort
> The educational value of being a good role model
> Respect for universal ethics including tolerance, generosity, unity, friendship, non-discrimination and respect for others.

All in all, the claim is that the goal of Olympism is to sport to promote the balanced development of people as an essential step in building a peaceful world society that places a high value on human dignity.

Pray tell me, therefore, where in the noble sentiments expressed above does it even intimate that a country ought to strive to "own the podium," that athletes are defending their country's honor, that they should feel shame if they did their best and didn't win a medal, or—say—that multi-millionaire National Basketball Association professionals ought to represent their country of origin at the Games!

What a travesty it has all become! Thank goodness that many fine athletes don't believe this tripe that has been visited upon us! However, the people do love a spectacle, and the 2000 Olympic Games held in Sydney, Australia, for example, were a spectacle from start to finish. Sydney, Australia evidently wanted worldwide recognition. Without doubt, Sydney got recognition! The world's outstanding athletes wanted the opportunity to demonstrate their excellence. From all reports they had such an occasion to their hearts' and abilities' content. The International Olympic Committee, along with their counterparts in each of the 200 participating nations, earnestly desired the show to go on; it went on with a bang!

Sydney spent an enormous amount of money and energy to finance and otherwise support this extravaganza and surrounding competition. The IOC and its affiliates remained solvent for another four years, while Sydney contemplated its involvement with this enormous event and its aftermath. "Problem, what problem?" most people in the public sector would assuredly ask if they were confronted with such a question.

The Problem

This analysis revolves around the criticisms of the "abolish the Games group" made by Sir William Rees-Mogg (1988, pp. 7-8) He is one of the Olympic Movement's most vituperative opponents. He believes the problem the problem to be of enormous magnitude then. I can only offer the firm opinion that somehow "enormous magnitude" has grown by "light years" since then. In 1988 he listed fifteen sub–problems in no particular order of importance except for the first criticism that sets the tone for the remainder: "The Olympic Games have become a grotesque jamboree of international hypocrisy. Whatever idealism they once had has been lost. The Games now stand for some of the things which are most rotten and corrupt in the modern world, for prestige, nationalism, publicity, prejudice, bureaucracy, and the exploitation of talent" (p. 7).

It would not be appropriate to enumerate here *in great detail* the remaining 14 problems and issues brought forward by Rees-Mogg. Simply put, however, he stated that "The Games have been taken over by a vulgar nationalism, in place of the spirit of internationalism for which they were revived" (p.7). He decried also that, in addition to promoting racial intolerance, "the objectives of many national Olympic programmes is the glorification and self-assertion of totalitarian state regimes," often "vile regimes guilty of many of the crimes which the Olympic Games are supposed to outlaw" (p. 7).

Rees-Mogg decried further "The administration of the Olympic Games [that] is politically influenced and morally bankrupt" (p. 7). Additionally, at this point, he asserted that "the international bureaucracies of several sports have become among the most odious of the world." In this respect he lashes out especially at tennis, chess, cricket, and track and field. Still further, he charges that threats by countries to boycott the Olympics have time and again made it a political arena akin to the United Nations.

The messenger has not yet completed his message. Rees-Mogg condemns "the worship of professionally abnormal muscular development," and states that it is "a form of idolatry to which ordinary life is often sacrificed" (p. 7). Since these words were written in 1988, these problems have assuredly not been corrected. They have actually worsened (e.g., ever-more drugs to enhance performance, bribery of officials assigned to site selection). The entire problem of drug ingestion to promote bodily development for enhanced performance has now become legendary. Couple this with over-training begun at early ages in selected sports for both boys and girls, and it can be argued safely that *natural*, all-round development has been thwarted for a great many young people, not to mention the fact that only a minute number makes it through to "Olympic glory." More could be said, but the point has been made. Basically, Rees-Mogg has claimed that it has become a world "in which good *values* are taken by dishonest men and put to shameful uses" (p. 8).

Social Forces as Value Determinants

In the present discussion about the Olympic Games, it may be worthwhile to first take a brief look at the "Olympic Games Problem" from the standpoint of the discipline of sociology. This is because in an analysis such as this, the investigator soon realizes the importance of the major social forces (e.g., values, economics, religion) as determinants of the direction a society may take at any given moment. Sociology can indeed help with the question of *values*. For example, Parsons' complex theory of social action can be used to place any theory of social or individual values in perspective. His general action system is composed of four major analytically separable subsystems: (1) *the cultural system*, (2) *the social system*, (3) *the psychological system*, and (4) *the system of the behavioral organism*. The theory explains how these subsystems compose *a hierarchy of societal control and conditioning* (Johnson, 1969, pp. 46-58; Johnson, 1994, pp. 57 et ff.).

The cultural system at the top in the action-theory hierarchy provides the basic structure and its components, in a sense, thereby, programming the complete action system. The social system is next in descending order; it has to be more or less harmoniously related to the *functional* problems of social systems. The same holds for the structure and functional problems of the third level, the psychological system (personality), and the fourth level, the system of the behavioral organism (i.e., the individuals involved). Further, the subsystem of culture exercises "control" over the social system, and so on up and down the scale. Legitimation is provided to the level below or "pressure to conform" if there is inconsistency. Thus, there is a "strain toward consistency" among the system levels, led and controlled from above downwards.

What is immediately important to keep in mind is that there are *four levels of structure within the social system* itself (e.g., Hong Kong as a social system within Southeast Asia and, more recently, in its developing relationship with Mainland China's culture). Proceeding from the highest to the lowest level– i.e., from the general to the more specific–we again find four levels that are designated as (1) values, (2) norms, (3) the structure of collectivities, and (4) the structure of roles. All of these levels are normative in that the social structure is composed of sanctioned cultural limits within which certain types of behavior are mandatory or acceptable. Keeping in mind for the present discussion that *values are at the top* —the highest level—and that there are many categories of values (scientific, artistic, *sporting*, and values for personalities, etc.). These social values–including *sport* values too, of course–are simply

138

assessments of the ideal general character for the social system in question. Finally, the basic point to keep in mind here is that *individual* values about sport will *inevitably* be "conditioned" by the social values prevailing in any given culture. In other words, there will be very strong pressure to conform.

Use of the Term "Value" in Philosophy

Moving from the discipline of sociology to that of philosophy, the investigator will use the term "value" as equivalent to the concepts of "worth" and "goodness." The opposite of these terms (i.e., "evil") will be referred to as "disvalue." It is possible, also, to draw a distinction between two kinds of value; namely, *intrinsic* value and *extrinsic* value. When a human experience has intrinsic value, therefore, it is good or valuable in itself—i.e., an end in itself. An experience that has extrinsic value is one that brings about goodness or value also, but such goodness or value serves *as a means to the achievement of something or some gain in life..*

One of the four major subdivisions of philosophy has been called *axiology* (or the study of values). Until philosophy's so-called "Age of Analysis" became so strongly entrenched in the Western world at least, it was argued typically that the study of values was *the* end result of philosophizing as a process. It was argued that a person should develop a system of values consistent with his/her beliefs in the subdivisions of *metaphysics* (questions about reality), *epistemology* (acquisition of knowledge), and *logic* (exact relating of ideas). Some believed that values existed only because of the interest of the "valuer" *(the interest theory). The existence theory,* conversely, held that values exist independently in the universe, although they are important in a vacuum, so to speak. They could be considered as essence added to existence, so to speak. A pragmatist (e.g., an experimentalist) views value in a significantly different manner *(the experimentalist theory).* Here values that yield practical results that have "cash value" bring about the possibility of greater happiness through more effective values in the future. One further theory, *the part-whole theory,* is explained by the idea that effective relating of parts to the whole brings about the highest values (Zeigler, 2010, p, 67).

Domains of Value Under Axiology

The study of ethics under axiology considers morality, conduct, good and evil, and ultimate objectives in life. There are a number of approaches to the problem of whether life, as humans know it, is worthwhile. Some people are eternally hopeful (*optimism*), while others wonder whether life is worth the struggle (*pessimism*). In between these two extremes there is the golden mean (*meliorism*) that would have humans facing life boldly while striving constantly to improve one's situation. In the latter instance it is not possible to make final decisions about whether good or evil will prevail in the world.

A second most important question under ethics is what is most important in life for the individual. This is a fundamental question, of course, in this discussion about human values in relation to the Olympic Games. What is the ultimate end of a person's existence? Some would argue that pleasure is the highest good (*hedonism*). One position or approach under hedonism in modern history is known as *utilitarianism*.. Here society becomes the focus, not the individual. The basic idea is to promote the greatest happiness for the greatest number in the community. Another important way of looking at the *summum bonum* (or highest good) in life is called *perfectionism*. With such an approach the individual is aiming for complete self-realization, and a similar goal is envisioned for society as well.

A logical progression following from an individual's decision about the greatest good in life is the standard of conduct that he or she sets for the "practice of living." A *naturalistic* approach would not have a person do anything that leads to self-destruction; self-preservation is basic. In the late 18th century in Germany, Immanuel Kant, known as an *idealist*, felt that a person should act on only what should be considered a universal law. Similarly, orthodox religion decrees that humans must obey God's wishes that have been decreed with a purpose for all humankind. *Pragmatism*, defined loosely, suggest a trial run in a person's imagination to discover the possible consequences of planned actions.

Continuing with this line of philosophic thought a bit further because of the obvious relationship it has to involvement with the Olympic Games in one way or another (i.e., as participant, official, coach, governing body member, advertiser, governmental official, what have you?), certain interests we develop are apt to guide people's conduct in life. Those who are too self-centered are egotistical (*egoism*), while those feel their life purpose is to serve others are called altruistic (*altruism*). Many would argue, however, that Aristotle's concept of the "golden mean" should be deemed best, a desirable aim for a person to fulfill with his or her life span.

There are, of course other areas of value under the axiology subdivision of philosophy over and above ethics that treats moral conduct (e.g., *aesthetics* , that has to do with the "feelings" aspects of a human's conscious life). Further, because there has been a need to define still further values in the life of humans, specialized philosophies of education and religion have developed, for example. This applies further to a a sub–department of the mother discipline of philosophy that has become known as sport philosophy. In sport philosophy, people would presumably make decisions about the kind, nature, and worth of values that are intrinsic to, say, the involvement of people in sport however defined.

An Assessment of the Problem

The problem, I believe, is this: Opportunities for participation in all competitive sport–not just *Olympic* sport– moved historically from amateurism to semi-professionalism, and then on to open professionalism. The Olympic Movement, because of a variety of social pressures, followed suit in both ancient times and in the present. When the International Olympic Committee gave that final push to the pendulum and openly admitted professional athletes to play in the Games, they may have pleased most of the spectators and all of the advertising and media representatives. But in so doing the floodgates were opened completely, and the original ideals upon which the Games were reactivated were completely abandoned. This is what caused Sir Rees-Mogg to state that crass commercialism had won the day. This final abandonment of any semblance of what was the original Olympic ideal was the "straw that broke the camel's back." This ultimate decision regarding eligibility for participation has indeed been devastating to those people who earnestly believe that money and sport are like oil and water; they simply do not mix! Their response has been to abandon any further interest in, or support for, the entire Olympic Movement.

The question must, therefore be asked: "What should rampant professionalism in competitive sport at the Olympic Games mean to any given country out of the 200+ nations involved?" This is not a simple question to answer responsibly. In this present brief statement, it should be made clear that the professed social values of a country *should* ultimately prevail–and they *will* prevail in the final analysis. However, this ultimate determination will not take place overnight. The *fundamental social values* of a social system will eventually have a strong influence on the *individual values* held by most citizens in that country, also. If a country is moving toward the most important twin values of equalitarianism and achievement, for example, what implications does that have for competitive sport in that political entity under consideration? The following are some questions that should be asked *before* a strong continuing commitment is made to sponsor such involvement through governmental and/or private funding:

1. Can it be shown that involvement in competitive sport at one or the other of the three levels (i.e., amateur, semiprofessional, professional) brings about desirable *social* values (i.e., more value than disvalue)?

2. Can it be shown that involvement in competitive sport at one or the other of the three levels (i.e., amateur, semiprofessional, or professional) brings about desirable *individual* values of both an *intrinsic* and *extrinsic* nature (i.e., creates more value than disvalue)?

3. If the answer to Questions #1 and #2 immediately are both affirmative (i.e., that involvement in competitive sport at any or all of the three levels postulated [i.e., *amateur, semiprofessional, and professional* sport] provides a sufficient amount of social and individual value to warrant such promotion),*can* sufficient funds be made available to support or permit this promotion at any or all of the three levels listed?

4. If funding to support participation in competitive sport at any or all of the three levels (amateur, semiprofessional, professional) is *not* available (or such participation is *not* deemed advisable), should priorities–as determined by the expressed will of the citizenry–be established about the importance of each level to the country based on careful analysis of the potential social *and* individual values that may accrue to the society and its citizens from such competitive sport participation at one or more levels?

Concluding Statement

In this analysis the investigator asks whether a country should be involved with, or continue involvement with, the ongoing Olympic Movement—as well as all competitive sport—unless the people in that country first answer some basic questions. These questions ask to what extent such involvement can be related to the social and individual values that the country holds as important for all of its citizens. Initially, study will be needed to determine whether sport competition at either or all of the three levels (i.e., amateur, semi-professional, and professional) does indeed provide positive social and individual value (i.e., more value than disvalue) in the country concerned. Then careful assessment—through the efforts of qualified social scientists and philosophers—should be made of the populace's opinions and basic beliefs about such involvement. If participation in competitive sport at each of the three levels can make this claim to being a social institution that provides positive value to the country, these efforts should be supported to the extent possible—including the sending of a team to future Olympic Games. If sufficient funding for the support of *all* three levels of participation is *not* available, from either governmental or private sources, the expressed will of the people should be established to determine what priorities will be invoked.

PART VIII
Where Should We Want To Be?

Status of Physical Activity Education
(including Sport)

I am seeking to make the case here that sound physical activity education including a competitive sport experience is good for all boys and girls as they grow up to adult status. However, we can't discuss this question intelligently unless the growth and development pattern of the child is fully understood. It is argued that boys and girls today are simply not rugged enough, that a majority of them are either obese or overweight, and that they are mistakenly being allowed to lead "soft and easy" lives. Although parents should be careful not to employ undue pressures to influence the young person, nevertheless the child's basic needs must be met if a desirable result is anticipated. It should be understood that there is much more to life than sport. In this effort to convince you my reader that youth should be guaranteed the best type of physical activity education experience, I offer a recommended "formula" for the average town or city to follow with their youth. A list of sound principles and criteria for program evaluation is included.

Some people seem to think that a normal, healthy youngster should be playing tiddlywinks most of the time, while others go so far as to encourage regional and national sport tournaments for elementary school boys and girls. Now they even have elementary school children running the marathon! One of the quickest ways to start an argument in Canada, for example, is to suggest that boys (and girls too!) shouldn't be involved in overly organized competition at such a tender age. In most of these arguments, the antagonists are generally raising their voices when they should be reinforcing their arguments!

It is simply not possible to discuss organized sport for children and youth intelligently unless we are fully aware of the entire pattern of child growth and development. For example, what is the physical growth and developmental pattern of a ten-year old? What are the characteristics of this age? Or to put it another way, what are his or her needs? What follows in Part VIII will help you answer these questions for yourself.

144

<u>What Do You Want for Your Child?</u> Your child and mine are of the utmost importance to you and me. We want to be certain that we are "doing right by them." It's all right if we have made mistakes ourselves and have been hurt by our errors. It isn't even too bad, if we continue to commit these bad habits in later life. But when it comes to our own children, that's a "horse of another color." If you want to find out what a person really thinks, take a look at what he or she is encouraging his or her own sons and daughters to do, and why.

<u>Are Boys and Girls Rugged Enough?</u> I believe that boys and girls today are simply not rugged enough. Our way of life has changed to such a marked degree that we are actually depriving our children of experiences that heretofore were commonplace. Time and again, children on the North American continent have demonstrated conclusively that their muscular strength and endurance is low. Translated into simplest terms, we are mistakenly "coddling" our children! Over 60 years ago, Dr. McCloy, State University of Iowa, arguably the top physical educator/scientist in the world for the first 50 years of the 20th century, warned that only one-fifth of the physical education classes in the schools at that time included enough exercise of a vigorous nature to contribute materially to an significant organic stimulation. (The situation probably hasn't improved down to the present for a number of reasons!) As far back as 1907, Dr. J. M. Tyler stressed that rigorous exercise of the fundamental trunk and limb muscles was absolutely necessary for the normal growth and development of the entire body. Despite these warnings, we have repeatedly ignored such advice, thereby demonstrating conclusively our forgetfulness of the fact that the human organism is far more body than "mind" (if it's even possible to consider them separately).

<u>Why Must the Child's Basic Needs Be Met?</u> Generally speaking, we all appreciate that the child (boy or girl!) at the age of 10 has certain basic needs which must be met to insure normal development. S/he needs an assured position in a social group. There should be adequate opportunity to develop bodily control, strength, and endurance. He needs organized games for a "team experience." He gains self-confidence, if he can excel at something. We should encourage good follower ship and cooperation as well as good leadership and competition. The child should be encouraged to exercise creativity in rhythms. Sufficient rest is imperative as are good food and plenty of fresh air. Although it seems to be especially difficult, we should

impress upon this youngster that good posture through correct movement and sitting patterns is actually the most comfortable posture.

Why Is Adequate Physical Development Important? From the mental hygiene standpoint as well, a child (or an adult) who is physically underdeveloped tends to develop a sense of inferiority, a fact that could affect his or her social responses in several different ways. From a completely practical standpoint, for example, a person without what should be considered a normal amount of muscle is more susceptible to fatigue than an individual with adequate musculature. A fatigued organism is simply not up to the burden of everyday life. Such a person is more apt to catch a cold or develop a minor infection. Much more serious is the fact that the flabby child or adult usually has a heart that is weak and not ready for emergencies. Here I am not necessarily thinking of the strain of a street attack or fight. It is more a question of the possible need to "battle" some infection like pneumonia. The late Dr. C. H. McCloy stated quite simply, "Adequate strength is good life insurance!"

What Environment Should a Child Have? What should parents do? This was the question my wife and I had in mind when we decided to move away from the city to the country. We wanted our children to grow up in an environment where they would have every opportunity to grow and develop normally. They roamed the fields. In the summer they swam in our dammed-up creek. They swung from the barn rafters and climbed the apple trees. Also, they played all sorts of sports and games without undue pressure.

At the same time we were most concerned that our children would profit from a well-rounded experience. They took music lessons and listened to good music. They took part in discussions and had various hobbies in which they collected coins, stamps, and what have you. From a physical recreational standpoint, our boy played various ball games and dabbled in archery, badminton, and table tennis. He fished in the creek, and he wrestled and boxed with his peers (and his Dad!) on a fairly regular basis.

A similar pattern was followed with our daughter. Once when she came home from summer camp, she had swum 100 miles, paddled 100 miles, and jogged 100 miles in 7 weeks! (Today she is in her early sixties and still has the motivation to stay fit through a planned exercise and endurance program.) Just recently she placed first in her age group in a cross-harbor swim/

When our son was 10 years old, I encouraged him to join a YMCA swimming team. (We followed the same pattern with our daughter, having started them both on swimming prior to entry into kindergarten.) He was definitely ready for a team experience, as long as the practices were not held too often. They were not so strenuous that his daily living pattern was disturbed. The amount of actual competition in meets should be carefully regulated as well. I knew that these principles were being followed by the team coaches (whose leadership in this YMCA was outstanding).

Lest you, the reader, think that I am trying to paint too rosy a picture, I want to reassure you that this boy was quite normal in all respects. He was noisy when eating; he was careless and sloppy with his personal belongings; he never remembered to brush his teeth unless reminded; he occasionally wet the bed when over-tired; and he seemed to revel in casual and slovenly attire!

<u>Why Certain External Pressures Should Be Avoided?</u> The point to be made here is that this was a child whose growth and development was following a certain pattern. His increase in height and weight was fairly steady. He needed plenty of nutritious food to encourage ossification of his skeletal structure in a normal manner. Permanent dentition was continuing. The small muscles were developing, and his manipulative skill was increasing. His posture had to be watched at this stage. His heart was developing less rapidly than the rest of his body, and its work was being increased. Fortunately, however, damage to the heart of a child (or at any age, for that matter) through exercise is typically avoided, because the skeletal muscles fatigue first. It is for this reason, obviously, that undue external pressures should not be brought to bear which would encourage a youngster to "fight on" indefinitely even though exhausted.

The boy of eight, nine, or 10 years of age has certain characteristics. He may well be sturdy, although he is often long-legged and rangy in appearance. He appears to have boundless energy and enjoys good health. He is developing a wider range of interests and a longer attention span. His goals are immediate, but he is learning to cooperate better. He is beginning to be interested in teams, and he is definitely more interested in prestige. This is the stage where sex antagonism appears, and girls are "vile creatures" to be avoided whenever possible. Although there are frequent lapses, the youth at this age is willing to assume certain responsibilities often begrudgingly.

Where Do Organized Sports Fit In? The short statement above covers only the growth and development pattern, with accompanying characteristics and needs, of one particular age group—the pre-adolescent boy. Naturally, there are many age groups in both sexes that the recreation director and the school sport and physical activity education professional should provide for at all times. There is no doubt but that competitive sport is playing an increasingly important role in our lives. Our problem, therefore, is to decided where organized sports fit into the total life style of people of all ages.

On the North American continent a definite pattern is readily discernible, one that can be analyzed by any reasonably intelligent, concerned individual. Our children and youth, not to mention a large percentage of adults, are fascinated (too much so!) by the idea of competitive sport. The anthropologist, the late Dr. Jules Henry, termed it accurately. People use sport as their "cultural maximizer (our community is better than your community, etc.). As a result, programs of organized competitive sport at all ages, which is usually for the few not the majority, appears at all levels of the educational system as well as in community recreational enterprises. This development is, of course, more true for boys and men, but sports and games for girls and women are now being offered similarly.

Why Competitive Sport Offers an Ideal Setting for Teaching and Learning? The late Harry Scott, of Columbia Teachers College, gave us much to think about in discussing the program of instruction in sport skills. He pointed out that the highly emotionalized situations in athletics, those "white-hot" moments when a decision to "do the right thing" should be made—offer the ideal setting for the teaching and learning of desirable social behavior to occur. However, he stressed that there is nothing inherent in such activity that guarantees that positive social learning will necessarily take place. He asserted that we must so organize our programs that this real-life drama of athletics will actually become a part of the general education of youth.

Why Should We Not Introduce Contact/Collision Sports Before Maturity? Up to now I haven't dealt with the matter of contact/collision sports for immature youth. From long personal experience, study, and observation, I can state unequivocally that I believe it is unwise (often indeed foolish and stupid!) to encourage violent, dangerous, "collision" sport to youth prior to physical maturity at, say, 14-15 years of age. (Even then I have my doubts about such sports as boxing, kickboxing, tackle football, and overly aggressive ice hockey where concussions are "rampant".) For that matter I would never encourage boxing or kickboxing competition, although properly supervised and outfitted boxing instruction might be desirable in an educational setting. On the other hand, carefully supervised, amateur wrestling can be profitably introduced in the late elementary and early high school days. I seriously question further whether today we can afford to equip adequately, to care for properly from a medical and physiotherapy standpoint, and to insure fully many of the high school tackle football teams that are sponsored in North America. (Interestingly, injuries seem to be considerably less in the vigorous sport of rugby despite the fact that expensive equipment is not needed.)

Where we often miss out as well in providing proper activities for youth also is in the matter of sound leadership and sportsmanship education. Since actions are conditioned by understandings and appreciations, it is necessary that all players be provided with guidance and instruction in personal conduct both as participants in, and spectators at, athletic contests.

<u>Why Should a Child Not Specialize Unduly</u>
<u>at an Early Age?</u>. My firm belief is that we should never encourage a boy or girl to become too narrow a specialist early in his or her sports career. I know this contradicts some of the "current wisdom" that only through early, intensive specialization can we hope to create the international gold-medal winner. Nevertheless, I contend that no athletic program for any school, community, state, province, or nation should exploit the young athlete. "Sport was made for people, not people for sport," asserted Dr. Arthur Steinhaus rightfully in mid-twentieth century. Conversely, we shouldn't encourage a young person to be a dilettante either, because the degree of organic vigor accruing to the individual is lessened when the purpose behind the participation is social recreation—and accordingly increased when the element of serious competition is introduced.

Where we often miss out as well in providing proper activities for youth also is in the matter of sound leadership and sportsmanship education. Since actions are conditioned by understandings and appreciations, it is necessary that all players be provided with guidance and instruction in personal conduct both as participants in, and spectators at, athletic contests.

<u>Why Should We Offer Youth More in Life Than Sport?</u> Despite this steady increase in competitive sport offerings, just about all of us would admit readily that there is, and should always be, more to life than sport. We are quick to criticize the young person who doesn't appear to be rounding into normal maturity. At a certain age we typically expect youth to become interested in the opposite sex, occasionally a mistaken expectation today—and develop heterosexual social recreational interests. We like to think also that young people are developing in other areas of recreational interest—in communicative interests such as conversation and discussion, as well as in writing; in learning interests that indicate a desire to know more about many aspects of the world that interest them; and in creative and aesthetic interests where the opportunity is afforded to create beauty according to individual appreciation of what constitutes artistic expression of form, color, sound, or movement.

However, I must state candidly that we can't state absolutely or precisely that such-and-such a program should be followed. Living one's life will always be (we hope) an art rather than a science. Nevertheless, we should proceed basically on the best available theory based on scientific findings. The opinions of educators, of medical scientists, and of social scientists point in a certain direction, of course, but often these conclusions are still based on inadequate evidence.

<u>Why Should We Guarantee the Best Type of Sport and Physical Activity Experience to Youth?</u> Despite this steady increase in competitive sport offerings, just about all of us would admit readily that there is, and should always be, more to life than sport. We are quick to criticize the young person who doesn't appear to be rounding into normal maturity. At a certain age we typically expect youth to become interested in the opposite sex—sometimes a dubious expectation today—and develop heterosexual social recreational interests. We like to think also that young people are developing in other areas of recreational interest—in communicative interests such as conversation and discussion, as well as in writing; in learning interests that indicate a desire to know more about many aspects of the world that interest them; and in creative and aesthetic interests where the opportunity is afforded to create beauty according to individual appreciation of what constitutes artistic expression of form, color, sound, or movement.

However, I must state candidly that we can't state absolutely or precisely that such-and-such a program should be followed. Living one's life will always be (we hope) an art rather than a science. Nevertheless, we should proceed basically on the best available theory based on scientific findings. The opinions of educators, of medical scientists, and of social scientists point in a certain direction, of course, but often these conclusions are still based on inadequate evidence.

Under What Circumstances Should We Criticize Those Who Sponsor Sports for Youth Too Quickly? If indeed adequate personnel, facilities, and programs are needed and, if "John Q. Citizen" doesn't fully appreciate this fact and is unwilling to see that these services are available, I believe it is grossly unfair and mildly despicable for anyone to automatically criticize those who would sponsor a variety of leagues and tournaments for youth. I would like to point out, however, that parents and school authorities should "either put up or shut up!" If parents want fine programs of sport, exercise, dance, and play for children and youth in the schools, the schools definitely have a prior claim to children for such programs during the school year! If the "enlightened citizenry" don't want these programs offered through the schools, they have a responsibility to provide these activities on an equal-opportunity basis through community recreation programs when the schools are not in session. If the public doesn't want to make these activities available either through the schools or the community recreation programs, it (the public) is simply stupid and ignorant and should somehow be enlightened. It is that simple, and yet that complex.

What Is a Suggested Formula for the Average Village, Town, or City? At this point let us be optimistic and prospective about this important matter. Accordingly, I would like to offer a "formula" that could well be tried out in communities of all sizes-and indeed is functioning in enlightened centers already. What I am recommending is steadily increasing cooperation between the recreation director and the physical educator/coach already. Basically, we know that boys and girls from eight to, say, 13 years of age are an interesting and challenging group with which to work. They are typically eager and anxious to try almost everything and anything. They respond readily to suggestion, and it makes us happy to see them at play (and occasionally "at work" too!).

As parents and enlightened citizens, we should encourage recreation directors to work more closely with school principals, the physical activity education supervisors (if your community is fortunate enough to have such people), and the high school physical activity educators and coaches. You may say that your community is already doing this to a degree. Nevertheless, I'll wager that not many communities have come up with this idea. Why not encourage the high school physical activity education men and women teacher/coaches to suggest "amateur coaches" for your teams from a leaders corps theu might recommend: young coaches of both sexes who would receive planned recognition and small honoraria for devoted, capable assistance. These young people might even join the education profession eventually.

Here, I feel, is our greatest potential for coaching leadership. I am certain that in most communities we are not making the best use of such an excellent source for young, interested leadership. Incidentally, along the way we could be running clinics for these young people to develop their leadership potential even further. Also, most of these young people are going to stay right in your community, and it would be useful to them and the community to encourage this idea of community service through an internship experience. Some of them might even go on to follow this type of endeavor as a profession.

Let's Ask Ourselves a Few Questions About Our Approach to Sport Sponsorship

Now, let's ask ourselves a few questions when we are contemplating the sponsorship of competitive sports programs for youth as follows:

1. Are we planning cooperatively with all concerned (the participant, the parents, the recreation director, the principal, the physical educator/coach, and local agencies)?
2. What values are we seeking for youth through the medium of competitive sports programming?
3. Are we placing sufficient emphasis upon the achievement of skills, cooperation, sportsmanship, and the enjoyment of the game?
4. Will the promotion of this activity result in the neglect of other boys and girls not sufficiently skilled to participate at this level?

What Is the Challenge of Competitive Sport?

Finally, here is the situation that all parents and community leaders face. The great challenge is—not to eliminate athletic competition for children—but to so employ the competitive sport experience that those inherent values for which we are all working will become a reality. I am not against competition for youth; I am against certain types of negative experiences in sport. We must work to achieve the available positive values through the agency of properly led, adequately equipped and housed, school and community sport programs. Sport is only worthwhile if it serves youth as a socially useful servant.

PART IX
Where Should We Be and How Can We Get There?

A Call for Professional Reunification

The placing of increased emphasis on their own profession of education is an important point for the physical activity educators/sport coaches today, because it is symptomatic of the many divisions that have developed in the past 50-60 years. Physical activity educators in the United States, for example, now recognize full well that there are indeed allied professions represented to a greater or lesser extent in the Alliance (AAHPERD). It is no longer a question of bringing these other professions back into the physical activity education fold; they are gone forever. However, in their own interest and that of physical activity education (including sport), they must be kept as closely allied as possible.

What is really crucial at the moment is that physical activity educators seek to bring about a recognizable state of **REUNIFICATION** within what is here being called the physical activity education and sport. If the present splintering process taking place is not reversed, both in the United States and in Canada, prospects for the future may be bleak indeed.

The profession must figure out the ways and means of unifying the various aspects of its own profession to at least a reasonable degree. Here the reference is to human movement, human motor performance, or developmental physical activity-however it is eventually defined—in exercise, sport, and related expressive movement for those who are qualified and officially recognized and officially certified in the theory and practice of such human movement—be they performers, teachers/coaches, teachers of teachers/coaches, scholars and researchers, practitioners in alternative careers, or other professional practitioners not yet envisioned.

To this point my position is that "we are not dead or even dying," because death implies complete inactivity. It could be argued that the field is presently quiescent, in that many seem to be following a "business as usual" approach characterized by (1) unimaginative programs, (2) routine drill with inadequate motivation, (3) too much free play even though inadequate skill levels prevail, and (4) teacher pedantry. With fifty states and commonwealths and ten provinces and three territories in Canada, and excluding Mexico (as we are prone to do typically) to consider on a continental basis, we simply cannot speak with authority as to the present state of what is called physical (activity) education generally, much less offer a specific, detailed analysis on a state-by-state or province-by-province basis. Therefore, we will take a different tack and listen for a moment to one of our severest critics, Harold VanderZwaag of The University of Massachusetts, Amherst. For years he argued vigorously that physical education has become an anachronism, that what it's all about is sport, dance, play, and exercise, all functioning quite separately within education and in society at large. What he suggested is "elimination of the field as such" (VanderZwaag, in Zeigler, 1982, p. 54). Where "it's at," he says, is "sport management!"

> (Note: Interestingly since Dr. VanderZwaag made that statement, there are now more than 250 academic programs in sport management in North America. However, as significant as this development has been in the provision of management personnel for competitive, commercialized sport, the emphasis accordingly has not been on developmental physical activity for normal, special, and accelerated populations. This is where the profession of physical education and sport should retain its place and identity!)

VanderZwaag's argument challenged physical activity education to define more carefully (or redefine) the very core of what it is all about when it requests space and time in the general education curriculum. Frankly, this is more than just a debate about terminology (e.g., the Germans have substituted the terms "sport" and "sport science" (*Sport und Sportwissenschaft*) for the former "physical education" (or körperlicher Erziehung). What knowledge, competencies, and skills are achieved through the medium of what has been called the physical education program for more than a century? It is useless to argue that other subject-matters haven't been this precise in making their case for inclusion in the curriculum. That's their problem; physical activity education and sport has its own that must be resolved very soon.

VanderZwaag's criticism and recommendation was not a completely isolated case. For example, consider the hypothetical case of a program called the department of kinesiology (or human kinetics) being eliminated from the leading university in a particular state or province. (Without singling out the state by name, this already happened, of course). For the past 30 years at least higher education has been in unusual difficulty financially. The extent of this hardship has varied from state to state and region to region. (The same problem came to Canada, but a bit later. Professionals in educational institutions often buy their own paperclips, staples, and stamps to do their own professional work.)

When university administrators have their backs to the wall financially, they obviously begin to look around for places to cut back arguing that only those programs central to the university mission can remain. If their glance happens to fall (1) on a department, unit, or division called "human kinetics," "kinesiology," or "sport studies" (formerly known as the physical education department), and (2) the undergraduate enrollment of this unit has been falling off, and (3) the many other arguments that can be mustered typically prevail, it is understandable that the rather desperate president or vice-president (academic) is going to think that human kinetics is one place where a considerable saving can be effected. "After all," he or she may argue, "there are six—or eight or 10 or 36!—other colleges and universities in the state turning out physical educators and coaches." Also, the quality of research in such units has often been questioned, arguably because they have been located in professional schools of education.

Further, this newly named department may also be "easy pickins," since it has relatively few tenured members, being completely separate from intercollegiate athletics and (possibly) intramural and recreational sports as well. In these activities (unfortunately typically designated as extracurricular), it is often the case that they are self supporting and can't be expected to provide much support to an academic unit that has not regarded them as being part of the department's basic structure.

Let us follow this hypothetical situation along a bit further because it gets to the heart of the problem of physical activity education and educational sport in a college or university setting. Members of the profession should be able to present a strong case for the support of a discipline that purports to examine "human motor performance in developmental physical activity in sport, exercise, and related expressive activities" within the academic program of the leading university in every state or province on the continent. It can be argued, also, that the field is unique, and that no other unit purports to have as its primary aim doing what it claims to do.

Further, since men and women must move in a great variety of ways in order to survive and to experience a desirable quality of life, it can be stated that it is essential to study this phenomenon in order to help people of all ages, be they normal, accelerated, or special-population individuals, to move with the greatest possible efficiency and with the maximum amount of pleasure and reward that comes from such movement. Additionally, it can now be argued successfully that lifetime involvement in developmental physical activity will actually help people live longer!

Steps That Could Well Be Taken

1. Problem situations such as those described above remind us that, first, if it is decided to change the name of a department (at whatever level of education), the basic terms offered for use should be fully understandable to people. (For example, there is the contested tale of a physics professor's reply to a plan to change a departmental name to "human kinetics." He stated, "Well, I suppose I shouldn't object too much if you want to call yourself by a term that is a subdivision of my field.") Interestingly, however, the word "kinesiology" has been in the dictionary for many years—but it never seemed to be used very much. However, the word "kinesiology" relates to all human movement, and there are many applied kinesiologists today in alternative medicine. As a result, the term requires delimitation for the purpose of physical education and educational sport.

2. The disciplinary unit in college and university circles is certainly best advised to strive for independent status (i.e., not under a school of education, perhaps under an arts and science division, but most desirably as completely separate, multipurpose division or unit within higher education. This is definitely better than following the "splintering pattern" that seems to be occurring so frequently at present. In such cases "small splinters are easier to excise," whereas units with basic physical-education instructional programs, professional education, and disciplinary-based programs, intramurals and recreational sports programs, intercollegiate programs, and programs in allied fields (e.g., health education) are harder to get at typically. There are so many *functional* cross-appointments.

3. The field is unwise to fight the idea that it has a hybrid status within higher education. By that is meant that it is not only a professional unit such as law is. It can also argue that it is a basic general education unit for all on campus (such as the subject-matter English), as well as being a department or division that can be regarded as a discipline because faculty members are seeking to add to the body of knowledge about human motor performance in developmental physical activity in exercise, sport, and related expressive activities. Because of this last very important point, the field must continue to

insist that all teachers/coaches in higher education be *scholarly* people. A university professor should be expected to generate and disseminate his or her knowledge in *either* so-called scholarly and/or professional journals (or clinics, textbooks, and monographs).

4. This brings up another important point that was touched on briefly above: professors of physical education and—say—kinesiology in universities would be well advised to *use their own terms* to describe what it is they are offering in our courses for students. If they persist in using course names like sociology of sport and exercise physiology, they are simply asking for future problems. Additionally, they have on their rosters typically a substantive block of professors who do not possess advanced degrees in these other disciplines, but who persist in identifying themselves as psychologists, physiologists, sociologists, historians, etc. If they feel that they *must* use the names of other disciplines, they should always put words like "sport" or "exercise" first. Better yet, use phrases like "functional effects of physical exercise" or "socio-cultural aspects of sport and exercise."

5. The field should publicize its willingness to serve the total community, including citizens of all ages within the political constituency that it has a responsibility for jurisdictionally. (In this connection, reflect on the incident of a track and field coach who was denied tenure by his dean because his publications were not refereed. Nevertheless, the outcry from the community and surrounding counties can still be heard. He received his tenure from a "higher level"!

6. Finally, on this important point of status, as true professionals in a field that has the potential to become an important profession (or series of allied professions), the field of physical activity education and sport has a responsibility to press for statewide or province-wide rationalization of its various program offerings so that equal opportunity will prevail for qualified citizens of all ages, abilities, colors, and creeds. To accomplish this, the field will have to join with colleagues and like-minded people wherever they may be found to implement lobbying techniques with legislators and other groups at all levels of society (Zeigler, 1990, pp. 9-10.

Looking to the Future

So "what is the problem," you might say. "If we indeed have made so much headway in the development of our body of knowledge, admittedly with significant help also from the efforts of those in our allied professions and related disciplines, why can't we just 'get on with it'?" This is a good question, but it also reflects our collective naiveté. As a profession we simply have not been able to "get in league with the future." We haven't even as a profession begun to officially recognize what the scholarly and scientific advances as explained above in the past three decades, much less what must be done to rescue us from the present doldrums in which we are reclining because of changing social conditions.

First, I believe that we must make a concerted effort to understand what futuristics or futurology is all about. The next step should be to apply these findings to one aspect of our lives—in this case, the possible future of the profession of physical education and educational sport. In Melnick's *Visions of the Future,* a 1984 publication of the Hudson Institute, three ways of looking at the future are suggested: (1) the possible future, (2) the probable future, and (3) the preferable future (p. 4).

As one might imagine, the *possible* future includes everything that *could* happen, and thus perceptions of the future must be formed by us individually and collectively. The *probable* future refers to occurrences that are likely to happen, and so here the range of alternatives must be considered. Finally, the *preferable* future relates to an approach whereby people make choices, thereby indicating how they would like things to happen. Underlying all of this are certain basic assumptions or premises such as (1) that the future hasn't been predetermined by some force or power; (2) that the future cannot be accurately predicted because we don't understand the process of change that fully; and (3) that the future will undoubtedly be influenced by choices that people make, but won't necessarily turn out the way they want it to be (Amara, 1981).

A variety of people have been predicting the future for thousands of years, undoubtedly with a limited degree of success.
Considerable headway has been made, of course, since the time when animal entrails were examined to provide insight about the future (one of the techniques of so-called divination). Nowadays, for example, methods of prediction include forecasting by the use of trends and statistics. One of the

most recent approaches along these these lines has been of great interest to me because I have been using a variation of this technique for more than 30 years with a persistent problems approach (originated by John S. Brubacher, 1947) leading to the analysis of our field (Zeigler, 1964, 1968, 1977a, 1977b, 1979, 1989, 2003). I am referring to the work of John Naisbitt and The Naisbitt Group as described in *Megatrends* (1982) and *Megatrends 2000* (1990). These people believe that "the most reliable way to anticipate the future is by understanding the present" (p. 2). Hence they monitor occurrences all over the world through a technique of descriptive method known as *content analysis*. They actually keep track of the amount of space given to various topics in newspapers—an approach they feel is valid because "the news-reporting process is forced choice in a closed system" (p. 4).

One of the "millennial megatrends" delineated by the work of the Naisbitt Group that appears to have significant implications for physical education and sport has been designated as the "Age of Biology" (1990, pp. 241-269). Explaining that biotechnology is rapidly becoming a powerful influence in our lives, Naisbitt and Aburdene stress that people should not be "somewhat put off by technology, and the confusing ethical component of biotechnology" because "the issues of biotechnology will not got away" (p. 242). The possibility of ultimately being able to manipulate inherited characteristics will have tremendous implications for the future as humans get involved in developmental physical activity in exercise and sport.

Melnick and associates, in *Visions of the Future* (1984), discuss a further aspect of futuristics—the question of "levels of certainty." They explain that the late Herman Kahn, an expert in this area, often used the term "Scotch Verdict" when he was concerned about the level of certainty available prior to making a decision. This idea was borrowed from the Scottish system of justice in which a person charged with the commission of a crime can be found "guilty," "not guilty," or "not been proven guilty." This "not been proven guilty" (or "Scotch") verdict implies there is enough evidence to demonstrate that the person charged is guilty, but that insufficient evidence has been presented to end all reasonable doubt about the matter. Hence a continuum has been developed at one end of which we can state we are 100% sure that such-and-such is not true. Accordingly, at the other end of the continuum we can state we are 100% sure that such-and-such is the case (pp. 6-7). Obviously, in between these two extremes are gradations of the level of certainty. From here this idea has been carried over to the realm of future forecasting.

Next, we have been exhorted to consider the "Great Transition" that humankind has been experiencing, how there has been a pre-industrial stage, an industrial stage and, finally, a postindustrial stage that appears to be arriving in North America first. Each of the stages has its characteristics that must be recognized. For example, in pre-industrial society there was slow population growth, people lived simply with very little money, and the forces of nature made life very difficult. When the industrial stage (or "modernization") entered the picture, population growth was rapid, wealth increased enormously, and people became increasingly less vulnerable to the destructive forces of nature. The assumption is that the comprehension of the transition occurring can give us some insight as to what the future might hold—not that we can be "100% sure." Yet at least we might be able to achieve a "Scotch Verdict" (p. 47). If North America is arguably that part of the world that is the most economically and technologically advanced, and will complete the Great Transition by becoming a postindustrial culture, than we must be aware of what this all means for our society. Melnick explains that we may have already entered a "super-industrial period" of the Industrial Stage in which "projects will be very large scale, services will be readily available, efficient and sophisticated, people will have vastly increased leisure time, and many new technologies will be created" (pp. 35-37).

It is important that we understand what is happening as we move further forward into what presumably is the final or third stage of the Great Transition. First, it should be made clear that the level of certainty here in regard to predictions is at Kahn's "Scotch Verdict" point on the continuum. The world has never faced this situation before, so we don't know exactly how to date the beginning of such a stage. Nevertheless, it seems to be taking place right now (the super-industrial period having started after World War II). As predicted, those developments mentioned above (e.g., services readily available) appear to be continuing. It is postulated that population growth is slower than it was 20 years ago; yet, it is true that people are living longer. Next it is estimated that a greater interdependence among nations and the steady development of new technologies will contribute to a steadily improving economic climate for underdeveloped nations. Finally, it is forecast that advances in science and accompanying technology will bring almost innumerable technologies to the fore that will affect life styles immeasurably all over the world.

The important points to be made here are emerging rapidly. First, we need a different way of looking at the subject of so-called natural resources. In this interdependent world, this "global village" if you will, natural resources are more than just the sum of raw materials. They include also the application of technology, the organizational bureaucracy to cope with the materials, and the resultant usefulness of the resource that creates supply and demand (p. 74). The point seems to be that the total resource picture (as explained here) is reasonably optimistic *if correct decisions are made* about raw materials, energy, food production, and use of the environment. These are admittedly rather large **"IFS"** (pp. 73-97). Kennedy (1993) also points out the difficulty "of international reform" in this connection as he writes of the "apparent inevitability of overall demographic and environmental trends" that the world is facing (p. 335).

Finally in this "forecasting the future" section, the need to understand global problems of two types is stressed. One group is called "mostly understandable problems," *and they are solvable.* Here reference is made to (1) population growth, (2) natural resource issues, (3) acceptable environmental health, (4) shift in society's economic base to service occupations, and (5) effect of advanced technology. However, it is the second group classified as "mostly uncertain problems," and *these are the problems that could bring on disaster.* First, the Great Transition is affecting the entire world, and the eventual outcome of this new type of cultural change is uncertain. Thus we must be ready for these developments attitudinally. Second, in this period of changing values and attitudes, people in the various countries and cultures have much to learn, and they will have to make great adjustments as well. Third, there is the danger that society will—possibly unwittingly—stumble into some irreversible environmental catastrophe (e.g., upper-atmosphere ozone depletion). Fourth, the whole problem of weapons, wars, and terrorism, and whether the world will be able to stave off all-out nuclear warfare. Fifth, and finally, whether bad luck and bad management will somehow block the entire world from undergoing the Great Transition successfully (pp. 124-129)—obviously a great argument for the development of management art and science .

What to Avoid in the Near Future

Transposing this approach to the future to the present situation of physical activity education and sport, and thereby to recommend what we *should do* in the years immediately ahead, we should undoubtedly give brief consideration to the question of *what to avoid* along this path (adapted from Zeigler in Welsh, 1977, pp. 58-59). First, there is evidence to suggest that we must maintain a certain flexibility in philosophical approach. This will be difficult for some who have worked out definite, explicit philosophic stances for themselves—especially those people who have positions that are extreme either to the right or left. For those who are struggling along with only *an implicit sense of life* (as defined by Rand, 1960), having philosophic flexibility may be even more difficult—they don't fully understand where they are "coming from!" All of us know people for whom Toffler's concepts of "future shock" (1970) and "third wave world" (1980) have become a reality. Life has indeed become stressful for these individuals.

Second, I believe that we as individuals must avoid what might be called "naive optimism" or "despairing pessimism" in the years ahead. What we should assume, I believe, is a philosophical stance that may be called "positive meliorism'—a position that assumes that we should strive consciously to bring about a steady improvement in the quality of our lives. This second "what to avoid" item is closely related to the recommendation above concerning flexibility in philosophical approach, of course. We can't forget, however, how easy it is to fall into the seemingly attractive traps of either blind pessimism or optimism.

Third, I believe the professional in physical activity education and sport should continue to strive for "just the right amount" of freedom in his or her life generally and in professional affairs as well. Freedom for the individual is a fundamental characteristic of a democratic state, but it must never be forgotten that such freedom as may prevail in all countries today had to be won "inch by inch." It is evidently in the nature of the human animal that there are always those in our midst who "know what is best for us," and who seem anxious to take hard-won freedoms away. This seems to be true whether crises exist or not. Of course, the concept of "individual freedom" cannot be stretched to include anarchy; however, the freedom to <u>teach</u> responsibly what we will in physical activity education and sport, or conversely the freedom to *learn* what one will in such a process, must be guarded almost fanatically.

A fourth pitfall in this matter of avoidance along the way is the possibility of the development of undue influence of certain *negative* aspects inherent in the various social forces capable of influencing our culture and everything within it (including, of course, physical education and sport itself). Consider the phenomenon of nationalism, how an overemphasis in this direction can destroy a desirable world posture or even bring about unconscionable isolationism. Another example of a "negative" social force that is not understood generally is the clash between capitalistic economic theory and the environmental crisis that has developed. The world must not proceed indefinitely with the idea that "bigger" is necessarily "better."

Fifth, moving back to the realm of education, we should be careful that our field doesn't contribute to what has consistently been identified as a fundamental anti-intellectualism (e.g., a coach mouthing ungrammatical platitudes). On the other hand, "intelligence or intellectualism for its own sake" is far being being the answer to our problems. As long ago as 1961, Brubacher asked for the "golden mean" between the cultivation of the intellect and the cultivation of a high degree of intelligence because it is need as "an instrument of survival" in the Deweyan sense (pp. 7-9).

Sixth, and finally, despite the ongoing and seemingly everlasting cry for a "return to essentials," and I am not for a moment suggesting that Johnny or Mary shouldn't know how to read or calculate mathematically, we should avoid imposing a narrow academic approach on students in a misguided effort to promote the pursuit of excellence. I am continually both amazed and discouraged by decisions concerning admission to undergraduate physical activity education programs made *solely* on the basis of numerical grades, in essence a narrowly defined academic proficiency. Don't throw out academic proficiency testing, of course, but by all means broaden the evaluation made of candidates by assessing other dimensions of excellence they may have! Here, in addition to actual ability in human motor performance, I include such aspects as "sensitivity and commitment to social responsibility, ability to adapt to new situations, characteristics of temperament and work habit under varying conditions of demand," and other such characteristics and traits as recommended as long ago as 1970 by the Commission on Tests of the College Entrance Examination Board (*The New York Times,* Nov. 2, 1970)

The Educational Task Ahead:
Developing a Quality PAE Program
(including Athletics)

The words "currently useful generalizations" may sound "anemic" in the description of what our program is all about within education at all levels. However, it seems much more practical and realistic to describe here what we generally accept as "our" responsibility" within the overall educational program. Hence, you will find concise summaries (i.e., "currently useful generalizations") concerning the management/administration of physical activity education (including athletics).

If this material seems reasonable, generally speaking, the credit should go to many of the administrators working in this area whose experience and insight has enabled them to gather and report a significant body of knowledge. Any deficiencies that may seem apparent when you attempt to apply these "generalizations" to specific problems may be caused by this author's inability to reflect correctly what many leaders have said and written, or by the peculiarities of the particular situation to which you are trying to apply them. The following statements may sound authoritative and definitive, but they must be challenged by you as you strive to apply them subsequently.

Consider the total physical education, and recreation program. It may be possible to suggest several additional categories, or to combine or eliminate some of the following areas that are recommended as a point of departure:

Aims and Objectives
Health and Safety Education (related)
Physical Education Classification
    or Proficiency Tests
The Required Program
Intramural Athletics
Interscholastic or Intercollegiate
    Athletics
Voluntary Physical Recreation
The Individual or Adaptive Program
Facilities and Equipment
Public Relations
General Administration
Evaluation

Aims and Objectives. The determination of aims and objectives seems basic. A philosophy of life should coincide with a philosophy of education. Thinking should be logical and consistent, and these beliefs should not conflict too much with practice in physical activity education (including athletics). Professional educators in this area should be operating on the basis of the "currently useful generalizations" for which they stand. If one calls principles "generalizations," this does not mean that he does not believe anything. It does mean that he/she will base actions taken according to what appears to be best at the moment.

(Note: for the remainder of this chapter to avoid awkwardness, I will use "he" instead of "she", but I trust the reader will understand that I am not thereby "downgrading" in doing so.)

It is most often practical to work from specific objectives toward general aims. Expediency may cause a physical activity educator to sidetrack some of his beliefs, but this does not mean that he must perforce lose sight of what he believes to be ultimately right. It is difficult for those in the field to agree on one basic philosophy. Obviously, there will always be at least several schools of thought. Although various beliefs should be expressed in a substantial way, truly definitive philosophies physical activity education (including athletics) are rare.

Although physical activity education has made a solid effort to achieve a stronger scientific base, science and philosophy have *complementary* roles to play in aiding the field to find its proper place in the educational system. Philosophy considers the *basic* problems of physical activity education (including athletics) in a systematic fashion. Philosophical thinking enables the professional worker to view his field as a whole. He will not see himself merely as an athletic coach, a physical conditioner, an organizer of intramural sports, or an athletic director.

Philosophy helps the professional to fashion a mental image of what his field should be. It is prospective in the sense that it forms a vanguard; it should lead actual practice. A philosophy, of course, must be practical, or it would be worthless. An instrumental philosophy would necessarily imitate science in part, but only as it serves as a plan for action. Science describes a field as it exists; philosophy pictures it as it should be. Philosophy is an excellent complement to science; it reaches and points toward the world of tomorrow.

A philosophy of physical activity education, typically as a part of an over-all educational philosophy, has a relation to the general field of philosophy. A prevalent view is that which holds a philosophy of life basic to a philosophy of education. To the former is assigned the establishment of fundamental beliefs; to the latter, their application to a specific field. A basic philosophy outlining specific aims and objectives could help physical activity education greatly and in many ways. This is true because there are now many serious conflicts dangerously splitting the field within education and "outside" in society at large. Yet all factions might readily agree that it is important for the administrator of physical activity education to strive to form a sound philosophy.

Health and Safety Education (Relationship to…). Physical activity education by its very nature is intimately related to the health and safety education program of an educational institution. Typically there are three aspects to the latter as follows:

Health Services. Health service today implies determining the student's health status, informing parents of any defects that exist, educating parents and offspring in the prevention of common defects, aiding the teacher to detect symptoms of illness, and helping to correct defects which are remediable.

It took many years for boards of education to realize that schools must be concerned with more than illiteracy. The new educational era demands that the school take unto itself practically all of the child's problems. Today, if conditions are ideal, the physician, medical specialist, nurse, dentist, psychologist, psychiatrist, nutrition expert, janitor, and teacher all have a part in the over-all job of keeping the child healthy.

Boards of education are increasingly taking the responsibility for health services. There are, however, many civic leaders who favor board of health control in this area. Cooperation between the two boards seems advisable on many occasions, but such an arrangement usually has its weaknesses. The fact that it is quite difficult for either agency to set policy which encroaches on the other's sphere of operation indicates that the responsibility for the health of the child should not be divided at this level.

"Medical inspection" was the now-archaic term formerly used for the medical examination of today. What is the school's responsibility for health appraisal? What type of medical examination should there be? Who should look after the correction of remediable defects? What is the relation of psychological services to the school health program? Who should maintain the health and accident records? What is the best plan for emergency care?

The medical examination itself serves more functions than is generally realized. In addition to diagnosis of defects and subsequent notification of parents, the school health authorities should strive to secure correction of remediable defects by careful guidance of the children involved. Each child must be helped to develop a scientific attitude toward bodily ailments. Having established the importance of the medical examination, ask your some questions about the actual examination the children receive. Is the parent invited to be present so that the physician can explain the results? Is the teacher present to learn more about the child for future guidance? Is the examination sufficiently complete and detailed? Too often, physicians are so rushed in the performance of their duties that the child receives only a more-or less perfunctory check-up.

It cannot be argued that a carefully maintained health record is superfluous in the development of a child. To be sure, limited budgets may restrict the adequacy of any such record. On the other hand, it is extremely important that the child receive the services of various educational experts. To get a complete picture of the child, youth, or young adult many things must be known about his environment, disease record, scholastic ability, social adjustment, and health practices. Health services should be involved with the appraisal, correction, and protection of children and youth throughout their years in the educational system.

Health Instruction. Health instruction is the second of three subdivisions of health and safety education. There are many questions to be answered here. Should health instruction classes be scheduled separately? What should a course in health include? What about the introduction of controversial subjects such as sex education? What should be the role of the physical educator in the field of safety education? Should driver education be included? Who should teach health-the physical educator, the health education specialist, a physician, or the science teacher? What attention should be given to mental health? Is a health coordinator necessary in a school?

The health instruction class has been a perennial problem. Facts about health have become a considerable part of the knowledge of how to live. Most important, of course, is that health education should be an influence in favor of "clean living." Although people know that regular medical checkups are advisable, they usually maintain their bodies in much poorer condition than they do their cars. Most people have their cars' oil changed regularly; yet, they insist upon waiting for pain before going to the physician.

Down through the years, health instruction has generally been taught somewhat poorly. Just as in the case of earlier "physical training," parents realized that health courses were, in many instances, next to useless. Even today they must still be convinced that most physical activity education teachers are anxious to incorporate the modem problem-solving approach into the teaching of health. Here is one area where the case method of instruction might be employed to advantage. Health instruction is more than just the teaching of principles and facts of healthful living; it is more than merely drawing the various systems of the body on the blackboard and explaining them superficially. Health education should have as its goal the integration of this book-knowledge with actual living achievement. This is no mean task-to motivate children and youth to use the facts to help them live at their best in order to be able subsequently to serve most.

Healthful School Living. Healthful school living itself can be subdivided into three categories: the conditions of the school environment, the conditions of the classroom experience, and the conditions of school organization. With so much school construction in all stages of development, the school building itself demands serious consideration. The taxpayer and parent must be shown that the demands of health and those of architectural beauty do not inevitably clash. And if they do, the students themselves should have first priority. The school plant must be *both* hygienic *and* beautiful if the student is to have the best educational opportunities. Although plans should be made for schools to be close to the geographical center of population, due thought should also be given to adequate size of building and surrounding area as well as to hygienic environment and the student's safety.

Conditions of the classroom experience are important, also. And what about the problem of discipline? Should the teacher dominate the students by sheer will power, or should the children be helped to develop their own standards of behavior? The end of all discipline would seem to be intelligent self-direction. Should such factors as undue fatigue, success and failure, noise and excitement, "sedentarianism", the hygiene of reading, and individual differences be considered?

The actual conditions of school organization play an important role in healthful school living. Is there a proper balance in the school among work, play, rest, and the taking of nourishment? For example, do we realize the educational potentialities of the school lunch by considering the adequacy of the cafeteria, time allowed for eating, economics of the project, student participation in conduct rules, and health supervision of the lunchroom employees?

Is the course curriculum properly divided, keeping in mind that the students are more efficient mentally in the morning? What supervision is there over the health of the individual teacher? Should the general tone of the child's day be "hurry"? Modern society is so rushed that a conscious effort should be made to slow down the daily tempo of the school program.

Physical Education Classification or Proficiency Tests. After the examining physician has informed the physical activity education teacher if the child is healthy, almost healthy, in need of adaptive work, or fit for only passive exercise, the teacher should test and classify the *normal* individual according to the objectives of the school's program. Testing and measuring are necessary in order to prove to administrators, supervisors, students, and the public that many students are physically and recreationally "illiterate." These tests provide classifications for the following purposes:

(1) To serve their individual needs.
(2) To promote fair competition between
    individuals and groups.
(3) To facilitate instruction.
(4) To assemble individuals of like interests as
    well as of like abilities.
(5) To insure continuity in the program from year
    to year.

A battery of physical education classification tests should include items that the department considers that most students should be able to pass within the time allotted by the school to physical education requirements. Every effort should be made to hold the tests used to the desirable standards of validity, reliability, objectivity, simplicity, standardization of procedure, duplicate forms, and "worthwhileness". Certain test items are often considered to be of greater importance to the development of the individual than others. If the student fails any part or all of the battery, he might be required to select activity in the order that the department feels is best for him.

For example, if a young man failed tests in swimming, body mechanics, motor fitness, leisure skills, and self-defense, he might be required to correct these deficiencies in the order that the department of physical activity education deems best. A similar battery of tests with differing emphases should be constructed for girls and women with priorities determined according to the department's stated philosophy. It is recommended that this philosophy should reflect the thinking of the best leadership in the field, educational administration, the staff of the physical activity education department, the parents, and the students themselves.

It might be wise to permit the incoming student to begin with some form of physical recreational activity, so that he will develop good attitudes concerning the continuing value of this type of activity. It is suggested that the activity he chooses coincide with some deficiency demonstrated by the classification tests.

The department should consider classification and proficiency tests in the following categories:

(1) Cardio-vascular efficiency.
(2) Age-height-weight.
(3) Motor fitness.
(4) Body mechanics.
(5) Self-defense
(6) Aquatics & life saving
(7) Dance
(8) Leisure Skills and appreciations.
(9) Health and sports knowledge.

Obviously, the work of the administrator/manager of physical activity education has only begun when tests have been selected and administered. When the tests have been carefully scored, rated, and appraised, the program needs of all the students can be evaluated. Testing can also aid in measuring the progress of the students and in grading.

The Basic Required Program.

    The conditioning program. If the student has not met the standards of the cardio-vascular and motor fitness tests, it is necessary to raise the general level of condition. Forcing an individual to follow a long, conditioning program, including such exercises as calisthenics, pulley-weight manipulation, rope climbing, and running, may frighten him away from physical activity education for many years to come. On the other hand, allowing the student to engage in any sport he desires may result in a continuation of the ineffectiveness displayed in the classification tests. It would seem logical to follow the middle road by selecting a combination of activities from each of these categories. The emphasis should be placed on motivating the student to participate with interest in all the phases of a complete physical activity education program based on sound health and safety education principles.

    The student's needs may be met best through the following activities:

    (1) General body-conditioning: through exercises, weight training, jogging, and swimming, and a course in body mechanics (if needed).

    (2) Aquatic activities stressing the development of an all-round ability in the water, including distance swimming, life-saving, water safety, stunts and skills, and water wrestling.

    (3) Tumbling and stunts.

    (4) Wrestling and self-defense instruction.

    (5) Sports participation of an individual, dual, and team nature stressing the acquisition of individual skills.

A conditioning program for a definite period of, say, six to twelve weeks might include activity in at least three phases of the above.

    The sports instructional program. A student showing a fair level of conditioning in the cardio-vascular and motor fitness tests might be referred immediately to sports instruction, but only for, perhaps, the first six weeks of the school year. With excellent instruction, interest can be aroused. In subsequent units, sports instruction can be coordinated with the other areas of instruction in which the student may have been shown to be deficient.

In the sports instructional program it is wise to schedule a yearly plan for all the various individual, dual, and team sports to be offered. A unit in a sports activity should be a planned sequence of learning and should take from twelve to thirty lessons for completion, depending on the difficulty of the activity. In planning a teaching unit, consideration should be given to the following:

> (1) objectives,
> (2) learning experiences,
> (3) subject matter, (4)
>   instructional methods,
> (5) a list of equipment and facilities needed, and
> (6) adequate means of evaluation.

The elective program. The elective program is actually a part of the physical activity education *requirement.* In this way it differs from the voluntary physical recreation program. "Elective" means that a student who has met all the standards set for the required program is permitted at some stage of the academic year (or perhaps for his total course) to select from suggested activities a physical education plan to suit best his needs and interests. Credit should be given for this activity, and definite instruction, supervision, and guidance should be offered, if it is to be considered a regular part of the course of study. If possible, the student should meet with an adviser to help determine the objectives of his program.

> Note: A department should give consideration to the question of a student maintaining proficiency in certain phases of the entire required program over the years (e.g., maintaining a minimum level of cardio-vascular conditioning).

Intramural/Extramural Athletic Competition. A fine intramural athletics program is most important in the achievement of a balanced overall program in physical activity education. Intramural athletics has improved significantly at the college and university level over the years. However, at the high school level the surface has barely been scratched. More help is needed in this area to fulfill the educational responsibility adequately. If the average student has a sound experience in competitive sports, he is likely to have a favorable "image" of physical activity education. High school boys and girls are the "public of tomorrow" that will decide whether physical activity education is worthy of financial backing at all levels of the educational system. Accepting as a premise the fact that competitive athletics is a desirable part of the total program, the intramural program provides recreational opportunity for leisure as well as another chance for the student to develop social contacts and group loyalties. As a result, the student should develop an appreciation of, and a lasting interest in, physical recreation. Healthful exercise and organic development must be considered as specific objectives.

> Note: Program administrators should keep in mind that "extramural athletic competition" may be desirable on selected occasions within the aegis of the Intramural Program. This would be separate and distinct from the varsity program.

Interscholastic and Intercollegiate Athletics. Interscholastic and intercollegiate athletics, along with intramural athletics, are integral to the total program. Under ideal conditions, participation provides the opportunity for fine educational experiences. The chairman or head of the department should be responsible for the program that should be financed by institutional funds. It is recommended that all gate receipts be placed into the general school or college fund. Unfortunately, there have been many problems in this aspect of the program to harass the administrator/manager. What is the present status of the interschool program? Are more stringent controls needed? What should be the principal's or dean's relationship to athletics? Are the health and safety of the participants being fully considered? Is insurance coverage adequate for any emergency? How should athletics be financed? What about the use of radio and television in athletics? What purpose do tournaments serve? Should a student be declared ineligible for competition because of poor grades in school work? Should more extensive athletic competition be encouraged for girls and young women? To what extent should interschool competition be encouraged at the elementary and junior high levels? What about professionalism, gambling, and the role of alumni? How should the program be evaluated? These are but a few of the questions that must be answered.

Because participation in athletics is entirely on an elective basis, it is a part of the program of voluntary recreation. Class credit in physical education should be given for team participation, however, but this should not take the place of the existing requirement. Team participation should never take the place of body mechanics instruction, self-defense instruction, aquatics, etc., unless duplication is involved (e.g., a member of the swimming team should not be required to take aquatics).

A student who falls below the normally acceptable academic standards of the institution might be asked to discontinue **athletics** just as he might be asked to discontinue other "extracurricular" activities. Each student's case should be considered individually. *All* sports are *major* sports. Each sport should have a varsity team with sound coaching. In colleges and universities, freshman teams should be operated with limited schedules involving very little traveling. This recommendation is based on the orientation needs of the freshman year.

Organized practice should be held only during the season in which the sport is played. However, for reasons of expediency and because football is a "unique phenomenon," spring practices in that sport may be held on the college/university level. However, they should be limited to a maximum of twenty sessions.

Coaches should be regular members of the school, college, or university faculty, with salaries and tenure similar to those of other teachers. Because of their ability as teachers in the sports they coach, the coach in higher education should be used as an instructor for these sports in the major program of the physical activity education department.

Voluntary Physical Recreation. This is the area in which the department can make a most lasting contribution. "Recreation assists man to become an artist in living." Physical recreation is that facet of the total recreational offering that relates primarily to the department of physical activity education and is so popular with children and young people. Physical activity educators have a responsibility to encourage students to develop healthy attitudes toward other areas of recreation-social recreational interests communicative recreational interests, aesthetic and creative recreational interests, and "learning" recreational interests. Often the "motor moron" is ridiculed, although he may be the class "brain" and an accomplished musician to boot. However, this individual is no more to be ridiculed than the proficient athlete who may be tongue-tied or confused when he is addressing a group. Both of these types are "more to be pitied than censured." Young people such as those described have both been exploited to a degree by either over-zealous, protective parents or thoughtless coaches. If "intelligent self-direction" is the aim of education, how truly uncultured both these young people are!

This judgment may seem a bit harsh, and it is possible that young people may not be happy at first exploring other facets of the recreational kaleidoscope. They can be helped to widen their activities, however, by example as well as by precept. When the athlete sees the coach enjoying himself in another sport or attending an art exhibit or a concert, he is likely to follow suit. However, teachers are often so busy providing recreational opportunities for others that they don't take time to enjoy recreation themselves. How should recreation education (i.e., preparation for future leisure involvement) be interpreted? Is recreation entertainment or part of the educational curriculum? What type of planning is needed to adapt school facilities for recreational purposes?

The Individual or Adaptive Program (Special Exercise Prescription). This phase of physical activity education for special-needs and children and youth is perhaps the most neglected. There is a definite need for this type of remedial work, although those who "control the purse strings" and/or administrators often do not feel it is important enough to merit a sufficient appropriation. This activity was once called *medical gymnastics,* and subsequently *corrective exercise.* The latter was shortened to *correctives.* This specialized area of physical activity education may well be called the individual program, the adapted program, adaptive physical education, or special physical education**. *(This is the ideal, of course. However, in today's world, it is the rare educational system that assists with this aspect of the ideal program.)***

Earlier studies show a very low percentage of normal posture among students. A very large percentage have rounding of the shoulders, while more than half of them have increased antero-posterior spinal curvature. There is an ongoing need for body mechanics instruction and corrective exercise. If physical activity educators do not help this situation in the formative years, the situation becomes almost hopeless toward the end of the high school experience. Obviously, this task is a matter that should be handled in a cooperative manner by physicians and physical activity educators.

Directors' ideas of health and correction are frequently very limited. Nevertheless, every administrator should recognize definitely what movements, techniques, and skills in their departments may have deleterious effects. They should remember that upwards of 75 percent of their students have faults in posture and consequently are using "bodily machines" that are out of correct alignment. The result is slow injury to joints, ligaments, and muscles. Hence, a basic need arises for fundamental corrective positions for all activities.

Even the posture of athletes is bad. Coaches and teachers should explain to athletes that their performance may be improved through normal joint alignment. This is, of course, most important at the elementary school level, where such rapid growth and "excessive discrepancies" in structural relationships occur. It should also be stressed that in addition to the possible benefits in health and physical efficiency, one's appearance will also be improved through normal joint alignment. From what has been said, it should be evident that the field of physical activity education must either do something about body mechanics and adaptive work or inform educational administrators and the public that it cannot do anything, or hasn't been allowed, or hasn't the facilities, or isn't interested in this phase of the work.

Facilities and Equipment. The question of adequate facilities and equipment for physical activity education is often a vexing one. Recommendations made in the past were often overlooked or modified to the point where the resultant facilities are not adequate for the task. Physical activity educators do not know all the answers about facilities and equipment. They could not possibly understand all of the engineering and architectural problems involved. They do understand, however, the problems they are likely to encounter after the gymnasium or the pool has been in use for some time. The task seems to be one of developing ways of forwarding such information to the attention of the architects involved in the planning.

Communities face almost insuperable odds in their attempts to finance education. This means that physical activity educators should be careful to avoid demands for unreasonable size in new gymnasia, locker rooms, and other facilities. With the tremendous growth in the school population, however, the needs cannot be underestimated, as these essential parts of a school building are going to be in use for a long time. Careful study and close coordination are necessary to insure that the public's money is spent to best advantage. When communities are short of classroom space, swimming pools that are going to be called "lakes" or gymnasia the size of airplane hangars are out of the question. Economy and adequacy are two words that may cause conflict unless the needs of physical activity education (including athletics) are made known in such a way that all concerned will appreciate the problems.

The question of combining an auditorium and a gymnasium is a perplexing issue. So-named "gymtoria" are certainly better than nothing, but in the final analysis they do not appear to be completely practical. Why the physical activity education program, on the one hand, or the variety of programs generally carried on in the auditorium on the other, should suffer from interruption is a question that is difficult to answer. Supplying both facilities costs a great deal of money, but formal education should not have to get along with inadequate facilities. (And don't forget that an "ongoing arrangement" with municipal recreation should be operative.) If physical activity educators work constantly to make their programs truly worthwhile, and sound public relations are carried out, the public is given a better idea of what the field is trying to accomplish. Under such circumstances, the money necessary to do the job should be forthcoming sooner or later.

Greater care seems to be needed in purchase and care of equipment. Money is easily wasted in poor planning and improper care of equipment. Equipment should be purchased locally to the greatest extent possible with the business being shared among the sporting goods stores in the locality. Asking for the submission of "tenders" is time-consuming, but such an effort to standardize equipment purchasing is highly desirable. A program should use quality equipment; yet, dealers should not be asked to forego a fair mark-up when they solicit school business. *Professional* physical activity educators should not expect "hand-outs" or prejudicial treatment simply because they control large equipment purchases.

A good "equipment person" is invaluable to a high school, college, or university. Careful storage of equipment is nothing more than common sense and good business. Proper procedures for the control and issuance of expensive equipment are highly desirable.

Public Relations. If this is an era of "new conservatism" because of the overall economic situation, physical activity educators must redouble their efforts to improve relations with the public. People are influenced more by actions than by what a group *says* it is trying to accomplish. Physical activity educators must be able to prove that children and young people are being helped to lead more effective lives through their participation in physical activity education. Although equipment and facilities in this area are at least as costly as those for any other subject area, the public will not complain *if it is given full value for its tax dollar.*

Although teachers and coaches are busy with their many duties, they should take the time to concern themselves with public relations. Very few people are aware of the various objectives of modern physical activity education. Physical activity educators (including coaches) still face the "aristocratic irresponsibility" of the traditionalists who would relegate them to the "frill" category. The public should know how much money is spent on intramural athletics for the *many*, as opposed to how much goes for interschool and/or intercollegiate athletics for the few. At the same time, the gate receipts of major sports should not be slighted. This money is a great help and is often used to finance intramural programs.

Continuous, reliable, responsible public relations will develop an informed public that will not mutter about "fads" and "frills." The administrator-manager of the physical activity education program should know what is news in his area and then make certain that it is presented to the various media in an interesting manner. Sports writers are allies in this venture; their influence is typically significant. A coach must be willing to devote some of his time to public speaking and must be adequately prepared when he/she speaks. A few basic talks about the various phases of the overall physical activity education program, including athletics, can be made to stretch a long way, but they must be developed with an eye to presenting the content of the message in the most entertaining manner.

Exhibitions and demonstrations of physical prowess and skill have been used often as public relations devices. Generally, these techniques are excellent, but they can be artificial and quite formal. To some, children must move like robots to show parents and the public that something is being accomplished in physical activity education periods. When this type of presentation takes place even some physical activity educators lose their sense of perspective. Rather than giving such stylized demonstrations, they might well present the actual teaching of the techniques that lead to proficient performance. This would be most interesting to parents, since it informs them of what happens in daily classes. Despite the various devices that are employed to further public relations, perhaps the best means of satisfying parents is to show them that their children are receiving as much individual attention as possible—and that they are progressing. A satisfied, happy student is the best "broadcasting station" that has yet been encountered.

General Administration. General administration is a sketchy area-a catch-all for problems that do not fit logically into any of the other subdivisions in this chapter. Administration or management of any educational program is the leadership of the personnel involved in conducting the program, and in that larger community of persons who are interested in, provide support for, and ultimately approve or disapprove of, the program itself.

Depending on how the task of an administrator is conceived, it can be simple or complex. If an administrator or manager is "the boss," matters will be quickly expedited. However, there may be a significant staff tum–over. On the other hand, if staff members are regarded as co-workers, much time may be consumed in discussing this or that phase of the program. However, in the latter situation the staff will be happier and may thus do a better job. On balance, there appears to be a logical middle path between dictatorship and anarchy that will result in optimum staff growth.

Relationship to the Teaching and Recreation Professions. Most people feel unable to devote sufficient time to carrying out their responsibilities in the many professional organizations whose functions often · appear to overlap. Many teachers have failed to fulfill their obligations here, thus making the burden heavier on those who are more conscientious. Professionals in the field physical activity education (including athletics) must take care not to forget their fundamental responsibility to the teaching profession as a whole. Allegiance is owed to the National Education Association, as well as to the American Association for Health, Physical Education, Recreation, and Dance. To promote the goals of general education, as well as to secure higher status for physical activity education, a much greater effort must be made in this area of professional service.

What about the relationship between physical activity education and the recreation profession? Cooperation among the various areas of recreation, parks, physical activity education, and athletics is highly desirable. The strength that can be gained from unity is enormous. Yet, often these groups appear to be "fighting for the use of the same bodies." If there are sharp differences between the activities inherent to the position of physical activity educator and that of recreation superintendent, an effort to determine a working relationship can be mutually beneficial. And what about the concept of the community school? This and many other questions wait to be answered through cooperative effort. The following analogy may help to clarify the entire problem. Both professionals in the final analysis are "playing on the same team"! The physical activity educator takes his turn as the pitcher quite early in the game, but not before the recreation director "pitches" to the preschool child. Sometimes the physical activity educator is batted out of the box very soon, and in many elementary schools he never gets beyond the warm-up stage. Under normal circumstances, the recreation director must pitch from the fourth inning on in this game that includes each player's entire life. Neither physical activity educator nor recreation director can forget that there are representatives of numerous other fields on this ball club: adult education, commercial recreation, private agencies, and others. Look to them for support and guidance. The status of the two professions, the physical activity educator as a professional educator, and the recreation director as a professional person, will grow as the worth of the overall program increases.

Evaluation. Many respected educators still say that there "is so little for the mind" in modern education, because they believe that misguided "John Deweyites" hold the fort. Careful scrutiny of school programs might give the opposite impression: "There is far less "for the body" in schools, colleges, and universities. Every year classification and proficiency tests indicate that students generally are woefully weak, misshapen, and uncoordinated. Evaluation is the subject matter of physical activity education is where many professionals falter. What is there to measure? If measurements were taken, whom would it influence? Only in relatively few schools are physical activity education grades figured in with "academic" averages. And, by the way, just what are we measuring?

Can we categorize the study of physical activity education an art, a social science, or a pure science? At present, it doesn't fit neatly into any category. The field was once one of the liberal arts, but in the Middle Ages it was torn from this lofty perch. Physical activity education appears to have deep roots in all three of the above areas depending on the angle from which it is viewed. One group stresses that it belongs to the humanities, because the aim is to help young people achieve certain attitudes and appreciations that will enable them to lead richer, fuller lives.

A second faction will say that physical activity education has a great role to play in the social sciences-that is, students are helped to acquire desirable personality traits through participation in various types of physical education activities. There is, certainly, a concern with society as a group of interrelated, interdependent people, but it is doubtful whether it is wise to be affiliated with the humanities in the sense that the field would serve chiefly as a discipline and as an instrument of factual knowledge only.

Those who emphasize the scientific attributes are anxious to gather as much systematized knowledge as possible through all possible avenues and types of research. In this, of course, there must be continual borrowing from mathematics and the physical sciences as well as the motor learning aspects of psychology. The present trend seems to be to make progress through statistics (i.e., proving right through a coefficient of correlation). Certainly there must be borrowing from everywhere possible in order to get all the facts needed.

Immediate concern about a high place for physical activity education in the curriculum hierarchy may help, but the aim should be to raise the physical fitness standards of *all* students—and ultimately of all citizens. Education "through the physical" is the correct slogan so long as rugged, healthy bodies for boys, girls, men, and women are the end result. The development of physical attributes belongs uniquely to the field of physical activity education. This should never be forgotten!

Major Processes to Achieve Desired Objectives and Goals

Without attempting to enumerate specifically where any stumbling blocks might loom in our path, the professions of sport and fitness and that of physical activity education should keep in mind the four major processes proposed by March and Simon (1958, pp. 129-131) that could be employed chronologically, as they seeks to realize their desired immediate objectives and subsequent long-range goals:

Problem-solving: Basically, what is being proposed here is a problem for the profession of (1) sport/fitness in the public sector and (2) physical activity education within education to solve or resolve. It must move as soon as possible to convince others of the worth of this proposal. Part of the approach includes assurance that the objectives are indeed operational (i.e., that their presence or absence can be tested empirically as the field progresses). In this way, even if sufficient funding were not available—and it well might not be—the various parties who are vital or necessary to the success of the venture would at least have agreed- upon objectives. However, with a professional task of this magnitude, it is quite possible, even probable that such consensus will not be achieved initially. But it can be instituted—one step at a time!

1. The Planning Phase. What is the best way to solve a problem? Initially I would recommend getting a small group of knowledgeable people together to figure out what the prerequisites are to getting started in the

direction of a solution. It may or may not be possible to get to the heart of the matter initially, but certainly the use of the familiar "questioning interrogative proverbs" can be brought to bear (i.e., the "who, what, where, when, why, how and how many" questions related to the problem).

At such an initial meeting it may be possible to come up with some tentative solutions for consideration and possible interim action that would keep the concern from developing even further. It may well be, also, that the "root causes" of the situation can be identified. Why, for example, wasn't the development of this issue or problem foreseen or anticipated? It is possible, also, that tentative solutions could be proposed at this first session for consideration at a subsequent meeting.

At a second, or follow-up meeting of the parties concerned, the group may be ready to select and validate some tentative, or even permanent actions of a corrective nature that might be taken. If several courses of action are recommended, they should be considered carefully and followed through theoretically with in-depth discussion. Finally, of course, one definite action should be proposed and adopted.

Concurrently, if it seems that problems or issues of this nature might be endemic in organizations of the type you are working in, it may well be that–looking to the future–selected, typical practices and procedures of the managerial system operative will need to be altered.

2. Persuasion: For the sake of argument, then, let us assume that the objectives on the way toward the achievement of long-range aims are not shared by the others whom the profession needs to convince, people who are either directly or indirectly related to our own profession or are in allied professions or related disciplines. On the assumption that the stance of the others is not absolutely fixed or intractable, then this second step of persuasion can (should) be employed on the assumption that at some level our objectives will be shared, and that disagreement over sub-goals can be mediated by reference to larger common goals. (Here the profession should keep in mind that influencing specific leaders in each of the various "other" associations and societies with which it is seeking to cooperate can be a most effective technique for bringing about attitude change within the larger membership of our profession everywhere.)

Persuasion strategies, or methods of social influence, are many and varied–legal, dubious, or illegal. In their popular book *The Art of Woo* (2007), G. Richard Shell and Mario Moussa present a four-step approach to strategic persuasion[2]. They explain that persuasion means to win others over, not to defeat them. Thus it is important to be able to see the topic from different angles in order to anticipate the reaction others have to a proposal.

> Step 1: Survey your situation. This step includes an analysis of the persuader's situation, goals, and challenges that he faces in his organization.

> Step 2: Confront the five barriers. Five obstacles pose the greatest risks to a successful influence encounter: relationships, credibility, communication mismatches, belief systems, interest and needs.

> Step 3: Make your pitch. People need a solid reason to justify a decision, yet at the same time many decisions are made on the basis of intuition. This step also deals with presentation skills.

> Step 4: Secure your commitments. In order to safeguard the long-time success of a persuasive decision, it is vital to deal with politics at both the individual and organizational level.

3. Bargaining. We will now move along to the third stage of a theoretical plan on the assumption that the second step (persuasion) didn't fully work. This means obviously that there is still disagreement over the operational goals proposed at the problem-solving level (the first stage). Now the profession has a difficult decision to make: does it attempt to strike a bargain, or do we decide that we simply must "go it alone?"

The problem with the first alternative is that bargaining implies compromise, and compromise means that each group involved will have to surrender a portion of its claim, request, or argument. The second alternative may seem more desirable, but following it may also mean eventual failure in achieving the final, most important objective.

We can appreciate, of course, that the necessity of proceeding to this stage, and then selecting either of the two alternatives, is obviously much less desirable than settling the matter at either the first or second stages. However, it doesn't seem that this is a situation where—in the final analysis!—bargaining (or haggling) can be ultimately accepted. How does one dicker about something so crucial to humankind's future? Nevertheless, there will inevitably be "stages along the way" as "official humankind" strives to serve its citizenry in the best possible manner.

4. <u>Politicking.</u> The implementation of the fourth stage (or plan of attack) is based on the fact that the proposed action of the first three stages has failed. The participants in the discussion cannot agree in any way about the main issue. It is at this point that the recognized profession has to somehow expand the number of parties or groups involved in consideration of the proposed project. The goal, of course, is to attempt to include potential allies so as to improve the chance of achieving the desired final objective. Employing so-called "power politics" is usually tricky, however, and it may indeed backfire upon the group bringing such a maneuver into play. However, this is the way the world (or society) works, and the goal may be well worth the risk or danger involved.

> Note: Obviously, the hope that it will not be necessary to operate at this fourth stage continually in connection with the development of the field within education. It would be most divisive in many instances and time consuming as well. Therefore, the profession would be faced with the decision as to whether this type of operation would do more harm than good (in the immediate future at least).

The Professional Task Ahead

As these words are being written, there is obviously a continuing value struggle going on in the United States that results in swings of the educational pendulum to and fro. It seems most important that a continuing search for a consensus be carried out. Fortunately, the theoretical struggle fades a bit when actual educational practice is carried out. If this were not so, very little progress would be possible. Based on recent reports worldwide, America needs to strive for improved educational standards for all. Renewed effort should result in the foreseeable future in greater understanding and wisdom on the part of the majority of North American citizens. In this regard science and philosophy can and indeed must make ever-greater contributions. All concerned members of physical activity education and allied fields in both the United States and Canada need to be fully informed as they strive for a voice in shaping the future development of their respective countries and professions. It is essential that there be careful and continuing study and analysis of the question of values as they relate to sport, exercise, dance, and play. Such study and analysis is, of course, basic as well to the implications that societal values and norms have for the allied fields of health and safety education, recreation, dance, and sport management.

Further, since men and women must move in a great variety of ways in order to survive and to experience a desirable quality of life, it can be stated that it is essential to study this phenomenon in order to help people of all ages, be they normal, accelerated, or special-population individuals, to move with the greatest possible efficiency and with the maximum amount of pleasure and reward that comes from such movement. Additionally, it can now be argued successfully that lifetime involvement in developmental physical activity will actually help people live longer!

Today, at the start of the second decade of the 21st century, we are beginning to truly understand the crisis in regard to the "fitness & health status" of the large majority of our youth. As I see it, the welfare of these boys and girls must be paramount. Competitive sport *within education* for the "accelerated" should really be promoted only after the welfare of all of our youth has been looked after adequately. (The professional sport management association [NASSM], celebrating its 25th anniversary in 2011, has a unique opportunity to exert some influence on the future of sport through their efforts in sport management education in the public sector of society.) Looking to this

186

end, I offer seven thoughts for consideration and possible approval:

1. I believe we need to truly understand "where sport has been" and "where it is now"—if we ever hope to know "where sport should go."
2. I believe sport, as a social institution, should be doing more good than harm.
3. I believe sport and physical activity management can be a fine profession under the right conditions.
4. I believe that the sport and physical-activity experience should be educationally and recreationally sound.
5. I believe there is a need for developing sport and physical activity management theory. The blossoming profession of sport should prove to the world that sport is or isn't doing what it purports to do.)
6. I believe, also, that we need an ongoing scientific inventory of "ordered generalizations about (a) what we know and (b) what we "think we know" about the "physical activity experience" in competitive sport (being careful to separate the "a" & "b" categories!).
7. I believe finally that we "had better be about our business very soon" with both pure and applied research.

These recommendations are made on the assumption that well-qualified teachers are available and have the opportunity within education to "do the job" as it should be done!.

1. That regular physical education and sport periods be required for all children and young people (who are presumably still in school) up to and including 16 years of age.

   (N.B. In the final two years of high school, personal fitness routines and elective leisure skills should be stressed.)

2. That human movement fundamentals through various expressive activities are basic in the elementary, middle, and high school curricula.

3. That physical vigor and endurance are important for people of all ages. Progressive standards should be developed from prevailing norms.

4. That remediable defects should be corrected through exercise therapy at all school levels. Where required, adapted sport and physical recreation experiences should be stressed.

5. That a young person should develop certain positive attitudes toward his or her own health in particular and toward community hygiene in general. Basic health knowledge should be an integral part of the school curriculum taught by qualified specialists in health and safety education.

> (N.B.: Note that this "common denominator" should be a specific objective of the field of physical activity education (including sport) primarily as it relates to developmental physical activity.)

6. That sport, exercise, and expressive movement can make a most important contribution throughout life toward the worthy use of leisure.

7. That boys and girls (and young men and women) should have an experience in competitive sport at some stage of their development.

8. That character and/or personality development is vitally important to the development of the young person, and therefore it is especially important that all human movement experience in exercise, sport, and expressive movement at the various educational levels be guided by men and women with high professional standards and ethics.

The Challenge to the Professional Educator

What I call the field of "developmental physical activity" practiced by professional educators in physical activity and related health education has never been more important in the helping of people of all ages and conditions to live both rewarding and longer lives. However, more than 100 years after courses began to appear in school curricula, we still find schools with good, bad, and indifferent programs. In many cases there is *no* program!

What, then, is the task ahead for professional educators? First, we should truly understand why we have chosen this profession as we rededicate ourselves anew to the study and dissemination of knowledge, competencies, and skills in developmental physical activity in exercise, sport, and related expressive movement. Concurrently, of course, we need to determine more exactly what it is that we are professing.

Second, as either practitioners, instructors involved in professional preparation, or scholars and scientists, we should search for young people of high quality in all the attributes needed for success in the field, and then help them to develop lifelong commitments so that our profession can achieve its democratically agreed-upon goals. We should also prepare young people to serve in the many alternative careers in sport, exercise, dance, and recreative play that are becoming increasingly available in our society.

Third, we should place quality as the first priority of our professional endeavors. Our personal involvement and specialization should include a high level of competency and skill under girded by solid knowledge about the profession. It can certainly be argued that our professional task is as important as any in society. Thus, the present is no time for indecision, halfhearted commitment, imprecise knowledge, and general
unwillingness to stand up and be counted in debate with colleagues within our field and in allied professions and related disciplines, not to mention the general public.

Fourth, the obligation is ours. If we hope to reach our potential, we must sharpen our focus and improve the quality of our professional and scholarly effort. Only in this way will we be able to guide the modification process that the profession is currently undergoing toward the achievement of our highest professional goals. This is the time—right now—to employ exercise, sport, dance, and play to make our reality more healthful, more pleasant, more vital, and more life-enriching. By "living fully in one's body," behavioral science men and women will be adapting and shaping that phase of reality to their own ends.

Finally, the recommendations for worldwide improvement of the status of the educational field that is called physical activity education (including extra-curricular sport) will not come easily. It can only come (1) through the efforts of professional people making quality decisions, (2) through the motivation of people to change their sedentary lifestyles, and (3) through dedicated professional assistance in guiding people as they strive to fulfill such motivation in their movement patterns. The mission in the years ahead is to place a special quality—a quality bespeaking excellence and dedication—in all of the professional endeavors of the field.

Finally, such improvement will not come easily; it can only come through the efforts of professional people making quality decisions, through the motivation of people to change their sedentary lifestyles, and through our professional assistance in guiding people as they strive to fulfill such motivation in their movement patterns These positive steps should be actions that will effect a workable consolidation of purposeful accomplishments on the part of those men and women who have a concern for the future of developmental physical activity as a valuable component of human life from birth to death.

Note: The information about the United States has been adapted from several sources, sections or parts of reports or books written earlier by the author. See **References and Bibliography** for Zeigler, 1951, 1962, 1975, 1979, 1988a, 1988b, 1990, 2003.

Part X
Counteracting America's "Western Value" Orientation

The term "*modernism*" is used to describe cultural movements in today's world that were caused by onrushing science, technology, and economic globalization. It is said to have started in the late nineteenth and early twentieth century. Conversely, *postmodernism*, as variously defined, can be described loosely as a late twentieth-century effort by some intelligent and possibly wise people to react against what is happening to this *modern* world as it "races headlong" toward an indeterminate future.

It can be argued reasonably that "The West's" thrust led by America is modernistic to the nth degree. To the extent that this is true, I am stating here that Canada—conversely—should work to counteract this value orientation as the world moves along in the 21st century. I believe that Canada can—and should do this—by adopting a position that might be called "moderate" postmodernism.

Granted that it will be most difficult for Canada to consistently exhibit a different "thrust" than its neighbor to the south and other leading Western nations. Nevertheless I believe that it is the time now for Canada to create a society characterized by the better elements of what has been termed postmodernism. In fact, I feel Canadians will be *forced* to grapple strongly against the basic thrust of modernism in the twentieth-first century to have any hope of also avoiding the "twilight" that is descending on "American culture" (Berman, 2000). You, the reader, may well question this stark statement. However, bear with me, and let us begin.

What is postmodernism? While most philosophers have been "elsewhere engaged" for the past 50 plus years, what has been called postmodernism, and what I believe is poorly defined, has gradually become a substantive factor in broader intellectual circles. I freely admit to have been grumbling about the uncertain character of the term "postmodern" for decades. I say this because somehow it too has been used badly as have other philosophic terms such as existentialism, pragmatism, idealism, realism, etc. as they emerged as common parlance.

In this ongoing process, postmodernism was often used by a minority to challenge prevailing knowledge, and considerably less by the few truly seeking to analyze what was the intent of those who coined the term originally. For

191

example, I am personally not suggesting, as some have, that scientific evidence and empirical reasoning are to be taken with a grain of salt based on someone's subjective reality. Further, if anything is worth saying, I believe it should be said as carefully and understandably as possible. Accordingly, the terms used must be defined, at least tentatively. Otherwise one can't help but think that the speaker (or writer) is either deceitful, a confused person, or has an axe to grind.

If nothing in the world is absolute, and one value is as good as another in a world increasingly threatened with collapse and impending doom as some say postmodernists claim, then one idea is possibly as good as another in any search to cope with the planet's myriad problems. This caricature of a postmodern world, as one in which we can avoid dealing with the harsh realities facing humankind, is hardly what any rational person might suggest. How can humankind choose to avoid (1) looming environmental disaster, (2) ongoing war because of daily terrorist threats, and (3) hordes of displaced, starving people, many of whom are now victims of conflicts within their own troubled cultures? Further, although it is still occasionally asserted, what rational being would argue that one idea is really as good as another?

What then is humankind to do in the face of the present confusion and often conflicted assertions about postmodernism from several quarters that have been bandied about? First, I think we need to consider the world situation as carefully as we possibly can. Perhaps this will provide us with a snapshot of the milieu to the point where we can at least see the need for a changing (or changed) perspective. The world needs a perspective that could possibly cause humankind to abandon the eventual, destructive elements of modernism that threaten us. An initial look at some of the developments of the second half of the twentieth century may provide a perspective from which to judge the situation.

Historical Perspective on the "World Situation"

In this search for historical perspective on world society today, we need to keep in mind the significant developments of the decades immediately preceding the turn of the twenty-first century. For example, Naisbitt (1982) outlined the "ten new directions that are transforming our lives." Then his wife and he suggested the "megatrends" they envisioned insofar as women's evolving role in the societal structure (Aburdene & Naisbitt, 1992). Here I am referring to:

1) the concepts of the information society and
   INTERNET,
2) "high tech/high touch,"
3) the shift to world economy,
4) the need to shift to long-term thinking in
   regard to ecology,
5) the move toward organizational decentralization,
6) the trend toward self-help,
7) the ongoing discussion of the wisdom of
   participatory democracy as opposed to
   representative democracy,
8) a shift toward networking,
9) a reconsideration of the "north-south"
   orientation, and
10) the viewing of decisions as "multiple
    option" instead of "either/or."

Add to this the ever-increasing, lifelong involvement of women in the workplace, politics, sports, organized religion, and social activism. Now we can begin to understand that a new world order has descended upon us as we enter the 21st century.

Moving ahead in time slightly past the presentation of Naisbitt's first set of *Megatrends*, a second list of 10 issues facing political leaders was highlighted in the *Utne Reader*. It was titled "Ten events that shook the world between 1984 and 1994" (1994, pp. 58-74). Consider the following:

1) the fall of communism and the continuing
   rise of nationalism,
2) the environmental crisis and the Green movement,
3) the AIDS epidemic and the "gay response,"
4) continuing wars (29 in 1993) and the peace movement,
5) the gender war,
6) religion and racial tension,
7) the concept of "West meets East" and resultant
   implications,
8) the "Baby Boomers" came of age and
   "Generation X" has started to worry and
   complain because of declining expectation levels,

9) the whole idea of globalism and
   international markets, and
10) the computer revolution and the specter of the
    Internet.

It appears that the world's "economic manageability"–or adaptability to cope with such change–may have been helped by its division into three major trading blocs: (1) the Pacific Rim dominated by Japan [now by China as well], (2) the European Community very heavily influenced by Germany, and (3) North America dominated by the United States of America. While this appears to be true to some observers, interestingly perhaps something even more fundamental has occurred. Succinctly put, world politics seems to be "entering a new phase in which the fundamental source of conflict will be neither ideological nor economic." In the place of these, Samuel P. Huntington, of Harvard's Institute for Strategic Studies, asserted that now the major conflicts in the world would be clashes between different groups of civilizations espousing fundamentally different cultures.

These clashes represent a distinct shift away from viewing the world as being composed of "first, second, and third worlds" as was the case during the Cold War. Thus, Huntington is arguing that in the twentieth-first century the world will return to a pattern of development evident several hundred years ago in which civilizations will actually rise and fall. (Interestingly, this is exactly what the late Arnold Toynbee in his now famous theory of history development stated. However, to confuse the situation even more, most recently we have been warned by scholars about the increasing number of clashes *within* civilizations!)

Internationally, after the dissolution of the Union of Soviet Socialist Republics (the USSR), Russia and the remaining communist regimes have been severely challenged as they sought to convert to more of a capitalistic economic system. Additionally, a number of other multinational countries are regularly showing signs of potential breakups. Further, the evidence points to the strong possibility that the developing nations are becoming ever poorer and more destitute with burgeoning populations resulting in widespread starvation caused by both social and ecological factors.

Further, Western Europe is facing a demographic time bomb even more than the United States because of the influx of refugees from African and Islamic countries, not to mention refugees from countries of the former

Soviet Union. It is evident that the European Community is inclined to appease Islam's demands. However, the multinational nature of the European Community will tend to bring on economic protectionism to insulate its economy against the rising costs of prevailing socialist legislation.

Still further, there is evidence that Radical Islam, possibly along with Communist China, is becoming increasingly aggressive toward the Western culture of Europe and North America. At present, Islam gives evidence of replacing Marxism as the world's main ideology of confrontation. For example, Islam is dedicated to regaining control of Jerusalem and to force Israel to give up control of land occupied earlier to provide a buffer zone against Arab aggressors. (Unfortunately, Israel is presently also building residences for settlers on land that by United Nations treaty was assigned to Palestine.) Also, China has been arming certain Arab nations, but how can the West be critical in this regard when we recall that the U.S.A. has also armed selected countries in the past [and present?] when such support was deemed in its interest?)

As Hong Kong, despite its ongoing protestations, is gradually absorbed into Communist China, further political problems seem inevitable in the Far East as well. Although North Korea is facing agricultural problems, there is the possibility (probability?) of the building of nuclear bombs there. Further, there is the ever-present fear worldwide that Iran, North Korea, and other smaller nations and terrorists will somehow get nuclear weapons too.

A growing Japanese assertiveness in Asian and world affairs also seems inevitable because of its typically very strong financial position. Yet the flow of foreign capital from Japan into North America has slowed down. This is probably because Japan has been confronted with its own financial crisis caused by inflated real estate and market values. Also, there would obviously be a strong reaction to any fall in living standards in this tightly knit society. Interestingly, further, the famed Japanese work ethic has become tarnished by the growing attraction of leisure opportunities.

The situation in Africa has become increasingly grim. Countries south of the Sahara Desert—that is, the dividing line between Black Africa and the Arab world—have experienced extremely bad economic performance in the past two decades. This social influence has brought to a halt much of the continental effort leading to political liberalization while at the same time exacerbating traditional ethnic rivalries. This economic problem has accordingly forced governmental cutbacks in many of the countries because of the pressures brought to bear by the financial institutions of the Western world that have been underwriting much of the development that had taken place. The poor are therefore getting poorer, and health and education standards have in many instances deteriorated even lower than they were previously. At this point one wonders how there ever was thought about the average family ever living "the good life."

America's Position in the 21st Century

Reviewing America's position in the 21st century may help us to get to the heart of the matter about where the world is heading. For example, we could argue that North Americans do not fully comprehend that their unique position in the history of the world's development will in all probability change radically for the worse in the twentieth-first century. Actually, of course, the years ahead are really going to be difficult ones for all of the world's citizens. However, it does appear that the United States is currently setting itself up "big time" for all kinds of societal difficulties. As the one major nuclear power, Uncle Sam has taken on the ongoing, overriding problem of maintaining large-scale peace. At the turn of the 20th century Teddy Roosevelt, while "speaking softly," nevertheless had his "big stick." The George ("W") Bush administration at the beginning of the 21st century had its "big stick", also, but it hasn't given a minute's thought to "speaking softly." The former president actually did claim that America's assertive actions are "under God" and are designed for the good of all humanity. This has caused various countries, both large and small, to speak out about many perceive as a bullying posture. Some of these countries may or may not have nuclear arms capability already. That is what is so worrisome.

America, despite all of its proclaimed good intentions, is finding that history is going against it in several ways. This means that previous optimism may need to be tempered to shake politicians loose from delusions, some of which persist despite what seems to be commonsense logic. For example, it is troublesome that despite the presence of the United Nations, the United States has persisted in positioning itself as the world superpower. Such posturing and aggression, often by unilateral action with the hoped-for, belated sanction of the United Nations, has resulted in the two recent United States-led wars in the Middle East and other incursion into Somalia for very different reasons. There are also other similar situations on the recent horizon (e.g., Afghanistan, the former Yugoslavia, Rwanda, Sudan, and Haiti, respectively). I haven't even mentioned the "Vietnam disaster" of the 1960s. And—let's face it!—who knows what the Central Intelligence Agency has been doing lately to make the world safe for American-style democracy. . .? Cuba first and now look out Venezuela!

There may be reason to expect selected U.S. cutbacks brought on by today's excessive world involvement and enormous debt. Of course, any such retrenchment would inevitably lead to a decline in the economic and military influence of the United States. However, who can argue logically that the present uneasy balance of power is a healthy situation looking to the future? More than a generation ago, Norman Cousins sounded just the right note when he wrote: "the most important factor in the complex equation of the future is the way the human mind responds to crisis." The world culture as we know it today simply must respond adequately and peacefully to the many challenges with which it is being confronted. The societies and nations must individually and collectively respond positively, intelligently, and strongly if humanity as we have known it is to survive.

Additionally, problems and concerns of varying magnitude abound. It seems inevitable that all of the world will be having increasingly severe ecological problems, not to mention the ebbs and flows of an energy crisis. Generally, also, there is a worldwide nutritional problem, and an ongoing situation where the rising expectations of the underdeveloped nations, including their staggering debt, will have to be met somehow. These are just a few of the major concerns looming on the horizon. And, wait a minute, now we find that America has spent so much more "straightening out" the "enemy" that its own debt has reached staggering proportions. The current financial xrisis has exacerbated this situation beyond belief...

In his highly insightful analysis, *The twilight of American culture* (2000), Morris Berman explains that historically four factors are present when a civilization is threatened with collapse:

1. Accelerating social and economic inequality,
2. Declining marginal returns with regard to investments in organizational solutions to socioeconomic problems,
3. Rapidly dropping levels of literacy, critical understanding, and general intellectual awareness, and

4. Spiritual death—that is, Spengler's classicism: the
emptying out of cultural content and the
freezing (or repackaging) of it in formulas-
kitsch, in short. (p. 19).

He then states that all of these factors are increasingly present on the American scene. Question: how did America get itself into this presenting highly precarious situation in regard to the daily lives of its citizens?

The Impact of Negative Social Forces Has Increased.

Keeping our focus on humankind's search for "the good life" in the twentieth-first century, in North America we are finding that the human recreational experience will have to be earned typically within a society whose very structure has been modified. For example, (1) the concept of the traditional family structure has been strongly challenged by a variety of social forces (e.g., economics, divorce rate); (2) many single people are finding that they must work longer hours; and (3) many families need more than one breadwinner just to make ends meet. Also, the idea of a steady surplus economy has vanished in the presence of a burgeoning budgetary deficit. What nonessentials do we cut from the debt-overwhelmed budget at a time like this to bring back what might be called fiscal sanity?

Additionally, many of the same problems of megalopolis living described back in the 1960s still prevail and are even increasing (e.g., declining infrastructure, crime rates in multiethnic populated centers, transportation gridlocks, overcrowded school classrooms). Thinking back to 1967, Prime Minister Lester Pearson asked Canadians to improve "the quality of Canadian life" as Canada celebrated her 100th anniversary as a confederation. Interestingly, still today, despite all of Canada's current identity problems, some pride can be taken in the fact that Canada has on occasion been proclaimed as the best place on earth to live. Nevertheless, we can't escape the fact that the work week is not getting shorter and shorter, and that the 1960s' prediction about society's achieving four different types of leisure class still seems a distant dream for the large majority of people.

Further, the situation has developed in such a way that the presently maturing generation is finding (1) that fewer good-paying jobs are available and (2) that the average annual income is declining (especially if we keep a steadily rising cost of living in mind). What caused this to happen is not a simple question to answer. For one thing, despite the rosy picture envisioned a generation ago–one in which we were supposedly entering a new stage for humankind–we are unable today to cope adequately with the multitude of problems that have developed. This situation is true whether inner city, suburbia, exurbia, or small-town living is concerned. Transportation jams and gridlock, for example, are occurring daily as public transportation struggles to meet rising demand for economical transport within the framework of developing megalopolises.

Certainly, megalopolis living trends have not abated and will probably not do so in the predictable future. More and more families, where that unit is still present, need two breadwinners just to survive. Interest rates, although minor cuts are made when economic slowdowns occur, have been reasonable. Yet, they had been inching higher until very recently. An unstable real estate market discourages many people from home ownership. Pollution of air and water continues despite efforts of many to change the present course of development. High-wage industries seem to be "heading south" in search of places where lower wages can be paid. Also, all sorts of crime are still present in our society, a goodly portion of it seemingly brought about by unemployment, drug-taking, and rising debt at all levels from the individual to the federal government.

The continuing presence of youth crime is especially disturbing. (This is especially true when homegrown youth turn to terrorism!) In this respect, it is fortunate in North America that municipal, private-agency, and public recreation has received continuing financial support from the increasingly burdened taxpayer. Even here, however, there has been a definite trend toward user fees for many services thereby affecting people's ability to get involved. Life goes on, however, but the question arises in ongoing discussions as to what character we seek for people within a burgeoning population.

What Character Do We Seek for People?

Functioning in a world that is steadily becoming a "Global Village," or a "flat earth" as described by Thomas Friedman, we need to think more seriously than ever before about the character and traits which we should seek to develop in people. Not even mentioning the Third World, people in what we call "developed nations" continue to lead or strive for the proverbial good life. To attain this state, children and young people need to develop the right attitudes (psychologically speaking) toward education, work, use of leisure, participation in government, various types of consumption, and concern for world stability and peace. If we truly desire "the good life," we somehow have to provide an increased level of education for the creative and constructive use of leisure to a greater percentage of the population. As matters stand, there doesn't seem to be much impetus in the direction of achieving this balance as a significant part of ongoing general education. We are not ready for a society where education for leisure has a unique role to play on into the indeterminate future? How might such a development affect the character of our young people?

What are called the "Old World countries" all seem to have a "character"; it is almost something that they take for granted. However, it is questionable whether there is anything that can be called a character in North America (i.e., in the United States? in Canada?). Americans were thought earlier to be heterogeneous and individualistic as a people, as opposed to Canadians. But the Canadian culture–whatever that may be today! –has moved toward multiculturalism quite significantly in the past two decades. Of course, Canada was founded by two distinct cultures, the English and the French. In addition to working out a continuing, reasonably happy relationship between these two cultures, it is now a question because of an aggressive "multicultural approach" of assimilating–as Canadians (!)–people arriving from many different lands. And let's not forget the claims of "first nations" whose 99 entities in British Columbia alone envisage more territory than exists!

Shortly after the middle of the twentieth century, Commager (1966), the noted historian, enumerated what he believed were some common denominators in American (i.e., U.S.) character. These, he said, were (1) carelessness; (2) openhandedness, generosity, and hospitality; (3) self-indulgence; (4) sentimentality, and even romanticism; (5) gregariousness; (6) materialism; (7) confidence and self-confidence; (8) complacency, bordering occasionally on arrogance; (9) cultivation of the competitive spirit; (10) indifference to, and exasperation with laws, rules, and regulations; (11) equalitarianism; and (12) resourcefulness (pp. 246-254).

What about Canadian character as opposed to what Commager stated above for America? Although completed a quarter of a century ago, Lipset (1973) carried out a perceptive comparison between the two countries that has probably not changed significantly in the interim. He reported that these two countries probably resemble each other more than any other two in the world. Nevertheless, he asserted that there seemed to be a rather "consistent pattern of differences between them" (p. 4). He found that certain "special differences" did exist and may be singled out as follows:

> Varying origins in their political systems and national identities, varying religious traditions, and varying frontier experiences. In general terms, the value orientations of Canada stem from a counter-revolutionary past, a need to differentiate itself from the United States, the influence of Monarchical institutions, a dominant Anglican religious tradition, and a less individualistic and more governmentally controlled expansion of the Canadian than of the American frontier (p. 5).

Seymour Lipset's findings tended to sharpen the focus on opinions commonly held earlier that, even though there is considerable sharing of values, they are held more tentatively in Canada. Also, he believed that Canada had consistently settled on "the middle ground" between positions arrived at in the United States and England. However, Lipset argued that, although the twin values of equalitarianism and achievement have been paramount in American life—but somewhat less important in Canada—there was now consistent movement in this direction in Canada as well (p. 6). Keeping national aims, value orientations, and character traits in mind as being highly important, of course, as well all of the material progress that has been made by a segment of the population, we are nevertheless forced to ask ourselves if we in Canada are "on the right track heading in the right direction?"

What Happened to the Original Enlightenment Ideal?

The achievement of "the good life" for a majority of citizens in the developed nations, a good life that involves a creative and constructive use of leisure as a key part of general education, necessarily implies that a certain type of progress has been made in society. However, we should understand that the chief criterion of progress has undergone a subtle but decisive change since the founding of the United States republic in North America. This development has had a definite influence on Canada and Mexico as well. Such change has been at once a cause and a reflection of the current disenchantment with technology. Recall that the late 18th century was a time of political revolution when monarchies and aristocracies, and that the ecclesiastical structure were being challenged on a number of fronts in the

Western world. Also, the factory system was undergoing significant change at that time.

As Leo Marx (1990, p. 5) reported such industrial development with its greatly improved machinery "coincided with the formulation and diffusion of the modern Enlightenment idea of history as a record of progress..." He explained further that this: "new scientific knowledge and accompanying technological power was expected to make possible a comprehensive improvement in all of the conditions of life–social, political, moral, and intellectual as well as material." This idea did indeed slowly take hold and eventually "became the fulcrum of the dominant American world view" (p. 5). By 1850, however, with the rapid growth of the United States especially, the idea of progress was already being dissociated from the Enlightenment vision of political and social liberation.

By the turn of the twentieth century, "the technocratic idea of progress [had become] a belief in the sufficiency of scientific and technological innovation as the basis for general progress" (Leo Marx, p. 9). This came to mean that if scientific-based technologies were permitted to develop in an unconstrained manner, there would be an automatic improvement in all other aspects of life! What happened–because this theory became coupled with onrushing, unbridled capitalism–was that the ideal envisioned by Thomas Jefferson in the United States has been turned upside down. Instead of social progress being guided by such values as justice, freedom, and self-fulfillment for all people, rich or poor, these goals of vital interest in a democracy were subjugated to a burgeoning society dominated by supposedly more important instrumental values (i.e., useful or practical ones for advancing a capitalistic system).

Have conditions improved? The answer to this question is obvious. The fundamental question still today is, "which type of values will win out in the long run?" In North America, for example, a developing concept of cultural relativism was being discredited as the 1990s witnessed a sharp clash between (1) those who uphold so-called Western cultural values and (2) those who by their presence are dividing the West along a multitude of ethnic and racial lines. This is occasioning strong efforts to promote "fundamentalist" religions and sects—either those present historically or those recently imported. These numerous religions, and accompanying sects, are characterized typically by decisive right/wrong morality. It is just this sort of "progress" that has led concerned people to inquire where we in the developed world are heading. What kind of a future is "out there" for humankind if the world continues in the same direction it is presently heading? We don't know for certain, of course, but a number of different scenarios can be envisioned depending on humanity's response to the present crisis of a society characterized by modernism.

Future Societal Scenarios (Anderson)

In this adventure of civilization, Walter Truett Anderson, then president of the American Division of the World Academy of Art and Science, postulates four different scenarios for the future of earthlings. In *The future of the self: Inventing the postmodern person* (1997), Anderson argues convincingly that current trends are adding up to an early 21st-century identity crisis for humankind. The creation of the present "modern self," he explains, began with Plato, Aristotle, and with the rights of humans in Roman legal codes.

Anderson argues that the developing conception of self bogged down in the Middle Ages, but fortunately was resurrected in the Renaissance Period of the second half of The Middle Ages. Since then the human "self" has been advancing like a "house afire" as the Western world has gone through an almost unbelievable transformation. Without resorting to historical detail, I will say only that scientists like Galileo and Copernicus influenced philosophers such as Descartes and Locke to foresee a world in which the self was invested with human rights.

Anderson's "One World, Many Universes" version is prophesied as the most likely to occur. This is a scenario characterized by (1) high economic growth, (2) steadily increasing technological progress, and (3) globalization combined with high psychological development. Such psychological maturity, he predicts, will be possible for a certain segment of the world's population because "active life spans will be gradually lengthened through various advances in health maintenance and medicine" (pp. 251-253). (This scenario may seem desirable, of course, to people who are coping reasonably well at present.)

However, it appears that a problem has developed at the beginning of this new century with this dream of individual achievement of inalienable rights and privileges. The modern self as envisioned by Descartes—a rational, integrated self that Anderson likens to Captain Kirk at the command post of (the original Starship Enterprise–is having an identity crisis. The image of this bold leader (he or she!) taking us fearlessly into the great unknown has begun to fade as alternate scenarios for the future of life on Earth are envisioned.

For example, John Bogle in his *The Battle for the Soul of Capitalism* (2007) argues that what he terms "global capitalism" is destroying the already uneasy balance between democracy as a political system and capitalism as an economic system. In a world where globalization and economic "progress" seemingly must be rejected because of catastrophic environmental concerns or "demands," the bold-future image could well "be replaced by a postmodern self; de-centered, multidimensional, and changeable" (p. 50).

Captain Kirk, or "George W" before "Obama", as he "boldly went where no man has gone before"–this time to rid the world of terrorists)–faced a second crucial change. Now, as the divided Obama American Government seeks to shape the world of the 21st century, based on Anderson's analysis, there is another force–the systemic-change force mentioned above–that is shaping the future. This all-powerful force may well exceed the Earth's ability to cope with what happens. As gratifying as such factors as "globalization along with economic growth" and "psychological development" may seem to the folks in Anderson's "One-World, Many Universes" scenario, there is a flip side to this prognosis. This image, Anderson identifies, as "The Dysfunctional Family" scenario. It turns out that all of the "benefits" of so-called progress are highly expensive and available now only to relatively few of the six billion plus people on earth. Anderson foresees this scenario as "a world of modern people relatively happily doing their thing–modern people still obsessed with progress, economic gain, and organizational bigness–along with varieties of postmodern people being trampled and getting angry" [italics added] (p. 51). And, I might add further, as people get angrier, present-day terrorism in North America could seem like child's play.

What Kind of A World Do You Want for Your Descendents?

What I am really asking here is whether you, the reader of these words, is cognizant of, and approves of, the situation as it is developing today. Are you (and I too!) simply "going along with the crowd" while taking the path of least resistance? Can we do anything to improve the situation by implementing an approach that could help to make the situation more beneficent and wholesome in perspective? What I am recommending is that the time is ripe for a country like Canada to distinguish itself more aggressively as being on a "different path" than "the West," dominated by the United States of America. To do this, however, individually and collectively, we would need to determine what sort of a world we (and our descendants) should be living in.

If you consider yourself an environmentalist, for example, the future undoubtedly looks bleak to you. What can we so to counter the strong business orientation of our society (i.e., being swept along with the "onward and upward" economic and technologic growth of American modernism)? Such is most certainly not the answer to all of our developing problems and issues. We should see ourselves increasingly as "New Agers" working to help Canada working to forge its own identity. I grant you, however, some sort of mass, non-religious "spiritual" transformation would have to take place for this to become a reality.

Let me offer one example based on my personal experience where I think Canada can make a good beginning in this respect. (Some who read this may wish to hang me in effigy [or literally!] for this assertion). Nevertheless I believe that Canada should strive to hold back the negative influences of America's approach to overly commercial, competitive sport in both universities and the public sector. At present we are too often typically conforming blindly to a power structure in which sport is used largely by private enterprise for selfish purposes. The problem is this: opportunities for participation in all competitive sport—not just Olympic sport—moved historically from amateurism to semi-professionalism, and then on to full-blown professionalism.

The Olympic Movement, because of a variety of social pressures, followed suit in both ancient times and the present. When the International Olympic Committee gave that final push to the pendulum and openly admitted professional athletes to play in the Games, they may have pleased most of the spectators and all of the advertising and media representatives. But in so doing the floodgates were opened completely. *The original ideals upon which the Games were reactivated were completely abandoned.* This is what caused Sir Rees-Mogg in Britain, for example, to state that crass commercialism had won the day. This final abandonment of any semblance of what was the original Olympic ideal was the "straw that broke the camel's back." This ultimate decision regarding eligibility for participation has indeed been devastating to those people who earnestly believe that money and sport are like oil and water; they simply do not mix! Their response has been to abandon any further interest in, or support for, the entire Olympic Movement.

The question must, therefore be asked: "What should rampant professionalism in competitive sport at the Olympic Games mean to any given country out of the 200-plus nations involved?" This is not a simple question to answer responsibly. In this present brief statement, it should be made clear that the professed social values of a country should ultimately prevail—and that they will prevail in the final analysis. However, this ultimate determination will not take place overnight. The fundamental social values of a social system will eventually have a strong influence on the individual values held by most citizens in that country, also. If a country is moving toward the most important twin values of equalitarianism and achievement, for example, what implications does that have for competitive sport in that political entity under consideration? The following are some questions that should be asked before a strong continuing commitment is made to sponsor such involvement through governmental and/or private funding:

1. Can it be shown that involvement in competitive sport at one or the other of the three levels (i.e., amateur, semi-professional, professional) brings about desirable social values (i.e., more value than disvalue)?

2. Can it be shown that involvement in competitive sport at one or the other of the three levels (i.e., amateur, semiprofessional, or professional) brings about desirable individual values of both an intrinsic and extrinsic nature (i.e., creates more value than disvalue)?

3. If the answer to Questions #1 and #2 immediately are both affirmative (i.e., that involvement in competitive sport at any or all of the three levels postulated [i.e., amateur, semi-professional, and professional sport] provides a sufficient amount of social and individual value to warrant such promotion), can sufficient funds be made available to support or permit this promotion at any or all of the three levels listed?

4. If funding to support participation in competitive sport at any or all of the three levels (amateur, semiprofessional, professional) is not available (or such participation is not deemed advisable), should priorities–as determined by the expressed will of the people–be established about the importance of each level to the country based on careful analysis of the potential social and individual values that may accrue to the society and its citizens from such competitive sport participation at one or more levels?

Further, as one aging person who encountered corruption and sleaze in the intercollegiate athletic structure of several major universities in the United States, I retreated to a Canadian university where the term "scholar-athlete" still implies roughly what it says. However, I now see problems developing on the Canadian inter-university sport scene as well. We have two choices before us. One choice is to do nothing about the "creeping semi–professionalism" that is occurring. This would require no great effort, of course. We can simply go along with the prevailing ethos of a North American society that is using sport to help in the promotion of social, as opposed to moral, character traits. In the process, "business as usual" will be supported one way or the other. A postmodern approach, conversely, would be one where specific geographic regions in Canada (the east, the far west. Quebec, and the mid–west) reverse the trend toward semi–professionalism that is steadily developing. The pressures on university presidents and governing boards will increase steadily. Will they have wisdom and acumen to ward off this insidious possibility?

The reader can readily see where I am coming from with this discussion. I recommend strongly that we take a good look at what is implied when we challenge ourselves to consider what the deliberate creation of a postmodern world might do for an increasingly multiethnic Canada. Despite the return to a Conservative minority government, expanding the elements of postmodernism in Canada has a fighting chance to succeed. In the rest of the world–especially the United States—forget it! Nevertheless, in its solid effort to become a unique, multicultural society, Canada may already be implementing what may be considered some of the better aspects of the concept of "postmodernism." For better or worse–and it may well be the latter–we are not so close to "the behemoth to the South" that we can't read the handwriting on the wall about what's happening "down there."

Can We Strengthen the Postmodern Influence?

My review of selected world, European, North American, regional, and local developments occurring in the final quarter of the 20th century may have created both positive and negative thoughts on your part. You might ask how this broadly based discussion relates to a plea for consideration of an increasingly postmodern social philosophy. My response to this question is "vigorous": "It doesn't" and yet "It does." It doesn't relate or "compute" to the large majority of those functioning in the starkly modern "North American" world. The affirmative answer–that it does–is correct if we listen to the voices of those in the substantive minority who are becoming increasingly restless with the obvious negatives of the modernism that has spread so rapidly in the modern world.

To help reverse this disturbing development, some wise scholars have recommended that the discipline of philosophy should have some connection to the world as it was described above. The late philosopher, Richard Rorty (1997), who was termed a so-called Neo-pragmatist, exhorted the presently "doomed liberal Left" in North America to join the fray again. Their presumed shame should not be bolstered by a mistaken belief that only those who agree with the Marxist position that capitalism must be eradicated are "true Lefts." Rorty recommends that philosophy once again become characterized as a "search for wisdom," a search that seeks conscientiously and capably to answer the many pressing issues and problems looming before humankind worldwide.

While most philosophers were "elsewhere engaged," some within the fold considered what has been called postmodernism carefully. For example, in *Crossing the postmodern divide* by Albert Borgmann (Chicago: The University of Chicago Press, 1992), it was refreshing to find such a clear assessment of the present situation. Time and again in discussions about postmodernism, I have encountered what I soon began to characterize as gobbledygook (i.e., planned obfuscation). This effort by Borgmann was solid, down-to-earth, and comprehensible. However, in the final pages, he veered to a Roman-Catholic position that that he calls postmodern realism as the answer to the plight caused by modernism. It is his right, of course, to state his personal opinion after describing the current political and social situation so accurately. However, if he could have brought himself to it, or if he had thought it possible, it might have been better if he had spelled out several alternative directions for humankind to go in the 21st century. (Maybe we should be thankful that he thought any one might be able to save it!)

With his argument that "postmodernism must become, for better or worse, something other than modernism," Borgmann explains that:

> [postmodernism] already exhibits two distinct tendencies: The first is to refine technology. Here postmodernism shares with modernists an unreserved allegiance to technology, but it differs from modernism in giving technology a hyper-fine and hyper-complex design. This tendency I call hyper-modernism. The alternative tendency is to outgrow technology as a way of life and to put it to the service of reality, of the things that command our respect and grace our life. This I call postmodern realism (p. 82).

At what point could we argue that the modern epoch or era has come to an end and that civilization is ready to put hyper-modernism aside and embrace Borgmann's postmodern realism—or any form of postmodernism for that matter? Can we hope to find agreement that this epoch is approaching closure because a substantive minority of the populace is challenging many of the fundamental beliefs of modernism? The "substantive minority" may not be large enough yet, but the reader may be ready to agree that indeed the world is moving into a new epoch as the proponents of postmodernism have been affirming over recent decades. Within such a milieu all professions would probably find great difficulty crossing this so-called, postmodern gap (chasm, divide, whatever you may wish to call it). Scholars argue convincingly that many in democracies, under girded by the various rights being propounded (e.g., individual freedom, privacy), have not yet come to believe that they have found a supportive "liberal consensus" within their respective societies.

My contention is that "post-modernists"—whether they recognize themselves as belonging to this group—now form a substantive minority that supports a more humanistic, pragmatic, liberal consensus in society. Yet they recognize that present-day society is going to have difficulty crossing any such postmodern divide. Many traditionalists in democratically oriented political systems may not like everything they see in front of them today, but as they look elsewhere they flinch even more. After reviewing where society has been, and where it is now, two more questions need to be answered. Where is society heading, and—most importantly—where should it be heading?

As despairing as one might be of society's direction today, the phenomenon of postmodernism—with its accompanying deconstructionist analytic technique affirming the idea that the universe is valueless with no absolute—brings one up short quickly. Take your choice: bleak pessimism or blind optimism. The former seems to be more dangerous to humankind's future that that of an idealistic future "under the sheltering arms of a Divine Father." Yet, some argue that Nietzsche's philosophy of being, knowledge, and morality supports the basic dichotomy espoused by the philosophy of being in the post-modernistic position. I can understand at once, therefore, why it meets with opposition by those whose thought has been supported by traditional theocentrism.

A better approach, I recommend, might be one of "positive meliorism" in which humankind is exhorted to "take it from here and do its best to improve the world situation." In the process we should necessarily inquire: "What happened to the "Enlightenment ideal"? This was supposed to be America's chief criterion of progress, but it has gradually but steadily undergone such a decisive change since the founding of the Republic. That change is at once a cause and a reflection of our current disenchantment with technology.

Post-modernists do indeed subscribe to a humanistic, anthropocentric belief as opposed to the traditional theocentric position. They would probably subscribe, therefore to what Berelson and Steiner in the mid-1960s postulated as a behavioral science image of man and woman. This view characterized the human as a creature continuously adapting reality to his or her own ends. Such thought undoubtedly challenges the authority of theological positions, dogmas, ideologies, and some scientific "infallibles".

A moderate post-modernist—holding a position I feel able to subscribe to once I am able to bring it all into focus—would at least listen to what the "authority" had written or said before criticizing or rejecting it. A fully committed post-modernist goes his or her own way by early, almost automatic, rejection of all tradition. Then this person presumably relies simply on a personal interpretation and subsequent diagnosis to muster the authority to challenge any or all icons or "lesser gods" extant in society.

Concluding Statement

In conclusion, it seems obvious that a *moderate* post-modernist would feel most comfortable seeking to achieve his or her personal, professional, and social/environmental goals through the stance that has been described. This position would be directly opposed to the traditional stifling position of, for example, "essentialist" theological realists or idealists. The world is changing. It has changed! These conflicting "world religions" are getting in the way of civilization's progress. The conflicts they cause could destroy humankind. A more pragmatic "value-is-that-which-is proven-through-experience" orientation that could emerge as one legacy of postmodernism would leave the future open-ended. That is the way it ought to be for the future on this "speck" called Earth in an infinite "multiverse"...

PART XI
Sport and Related Physical Activity in a Postmodern World

We have arrived at Part XI, the final one in this book. In Part I, I asked the question: Where in the world are we?" I was referring to (1) the situation in competitive sport in the developed world and (2) the situation in regard to physical activity education that presumably should be part of the educational curriculum at the elementary and secondary levels of education at least. As you appreciate, I have sought to explain progressively throughout this book how North America–along with the rest of the "developed Western world" following on its heels to a greater or lesser extent–has reached the point where the following conditions prevail:

(1) a very small percentage of youth and young adults gets involved regularly as "varsity athletes" representing their school, university, province, state, or country in some local, state, regional, or international competition; and

(2) the overwhelming majority of their fellow students, including special-need students are receiving good, fair, poor, or no physical activity education including intramural sport competition. (The assumption is that those in the #2 category should also be getting related health and safety education at all educational levels.)

This situation is replicated for out-of-school young adults and then continues on typically throughout people's lives until their death. This is not to say that opportunities are not made available for young, out-of-school adults who wish to "get involved," but such involvement is often expensive, inconvenient, difficult, and/or boring. *Additionally, citizens of all ages, including youth, are urged regularly to pay money in some form or another to watch "sport stars" compete in a variety of so-called gate-receipt sports.* This realm where "spectatoritis reigns" has grown almost exponentially during the second half of the 20th century with burgeoning professional sport and the Olympic extravaganza in its many and varied forms!

(Note: Interestingly, but sadly, a similar situation prevails with young people who have all sorts of "special needs." For example, we send "wheelchair athletes" to their own Olympic Games, but the Creator alone knows what type of

212

recreational sport is being made available for 99% plus of
people of all ages who are "wheelchair bound".)

Negative Forces Impacting Our Lives

While the above conditions have been evolving, we all appreciate the
significant developments that have transformed our lives in what has been
called "the emerging postmodern age." There have been many negative
social forces impacting upon our lives in various ways, and the problems of
megalopolis have not yet been solved to the satisfaction of many. Savants ask
about "the character" we are seeking for people, and daily people in one way
or another wonder whether "civilization" will ever achieve what was termed
"The Enlightenment Ideal."

The eighteenth-century movement of intellectual change that held so
much promise for humankind to be involved socially and politically in the
achievement of an ideal society seems still to be a distant ideal. To be sure,
many do have the opportunity to use their own reason to help with the
development of a superior type of state in those places where such input may
eventually contribute to the ideal world community. Yet today conflicting
hoary religions are still creating many seemingly insoluble problems that
threaten future life on our tiny planet.

World society is obviously in a precarious state. It is therefore
important to view present social conditions globally. Throughout this volume
I will be emphasizing that competitive sport has developed to a point where it
has worldwide impact, and also human physical activity should be so
organized and administered that it truly makes a contribution to what Glasser
(1972) identified as "Civilized Identify Society"–a state in which the concerns
of humans will again focus on such concepts as 'self-identity,' 'self-expression,'
and 'cooperation.'

To this point we know that we are organisms, living creatures, who
have reached a stage of development where we "know that something has
happened, is continuing to happen, and will evidently continue to happen."
However, underlying my entire analysis I am searching for the answers to *two
historical questions*: First, did humans in earlier times, equipped with their
coalescing genes and evolving **memes,** enjoy to any significant degree what
discerning people today might define as "quality living?"

(Note: Memes are sets of "cultural instructions" passed on from one generation to the next; see below, also.)

Second, did earlier humans have an opportunity for freely chosen, beneficial physical activity in sport, exercise, play, and dance of sufficient quality and quantity to contribute to the quality of life (as viewed possible by selected sport philosophers today)?

(Note: Of course, the phrasing of these questions—whether humans in earlier societies enjoyed quality living, including fine types of developmental physical activity—is no doubt presumptuous. It reminds one of the comedian whose stock question in response to his foil who challenged the truth of the zany experiences his friend typically reported: "Vas you dere, Sharlie?")

Can Humans Be Both "Judge and Jury"?

What makes a question about the quality of life in earlier times doubly difficult, of course, is whether present-day humans can be both judge and jury in such a debate. On what basis can we decide, for example, whether any social progress has indeed been made such that would permit resolution of such a concept as "quality living" including a modicum of "ideal sport competition" or "purposeful physical activity and related health education."?

There has been progression, of course, but how can we assume that change is indeed progress? It may be acceptable as a human criterion of progress to say that we are coming closer to approximating the good and the solid accomplishments that we think humans should have achieved both including what might be termed "the finest type" of sport competition.

In Part III, after calling the development of humans on Earth an "adventure," the question was raised as to whether human nature was predetermined or whether it is evolving. I explained that humans really weren't very sure about their "human nature" yet, and that there have been at least seven rival theories as to its essence extending from Plato to Freud more or less in the Western World—*not forgetting Lorenz's theory that humans are innately aggressive.*

There has been progression, of course, but how can we assume that change is indeed progress? It may be acceptable as a human criterion of progress to say that we are coming closer to approximating the good and the solid accomplishments that we think humans should have achieved both including what might be termed "the finest type" of sport competition.

One realizes immediately, also, that any assessment of the quality of life in prerecorded history, including the possible role of competitive sporting in that experience, must be a dubious evaluation at best. However, I was intrigued by the work of Herbert Muller who has written so insightfully about the struggle for freedom in human history. I was impressed, also, by his belief that recorded history has displayed a "tragic sense" of life. Whereas the philosopher Hobbes (1588-1679) stated in his *De Homine* that very early humans existed in an anarchically individualistic state of nature in which life was "solitary, poor, nasty, brutish, and short," Muller (1961) argued in rebuttal that it "might have been poor and short enough, but that it was never solitary or simply brutish" (p. 6).

Accordingly, Muller's approach to history is "in the spirit of the great tragic poets, a spirit of reverence and or irony, and is based on the assumption that the tragic sense of life is not only the profoundest but the most pertinent for an understanding of both past and present" (1952, p. vii). The rationalization for his
"tragic" view is simply that the drama of human history has truly been characterized by high tragedy in the Aristotelian sense. As he states, "All the mighty civilizations of the past have fallen, because of tragic flaws; as we are enthralled by any Golden Age we must always add that it did not last, it did not do" (p. vii).

America's "Golden Age"?

This made me wonder whether the 20th century of the modern era might turn out to be the "Golden Age" of the United States. This may be true because so many misgivings are developing about former blind optimism concerning history's malleability and compatibility in keeping with American ideals. As Heilbroner (1960) explained in his 'future as history' concept, America's still-prevalent belief in a personal "deity of history" may be short-lived in the 21st century. Arguing that technological, political, and economic forces are "bringing about a closing of our historic future," he emphasized the need to search for a greatly improved "common denominator of values" (p. 178).

However, all of this could be an oversimplification, because even the concept of 'civilization' is literally a relative newcomer on the world scene. Recall that Arnold Toynbee (1947) came to a quite simple conclusion about human development is his monumental *A study of history*—that humankind must return to the one true God from whom it has gradually but steadily fallen away. An outdated concept, you might say, but there is a faint possibility that Toynbee may turn out to be right. However, we on this Earth dare not put all of our eggs in that one basket. We had best try to use our heads as intelligently and wisely as possible as we get on with striving to make the world as effective and efficient—and as replete with good, as opposed to evil, as we possibly can.

Five Steps to Problem-Solving

In Part IV I looked starkly at the status of physical activity education and competitive sport in America (the United States primarily). I explained specifically how it developed historically that we got our priorities "all screwed up" in relation to both competitive sport and physical activity education and related health and safety education.

Then, on the assumption that society would want to solve any serious problem, I outlined five steps that society ought to go through as it sought to do just that beginning with "Where are we now? I ended with "What *exactly* (specifically!) should we do?" I averred that all children and youth need understanding of, and experience with, the following selected competencies:

1) *Correct body mechanics*
2) *Maintenance of physical fitness (cardio-respiratory and strength activities)*
3) *"Aquatic competence" (how to swim and elementary lifesaving)*
4) *An indoor & an outdoor leisure skill (e.g., badminton, tennis, golf)*
5) *A self-defense activity (major emphasis on defense…)*
6) *A aesthetic movement activity (e.g., social dance)*

Assuming that a number of people would not automatically rush to the telephone or computer to let their elected representative know what some "senior citizen" of physical activity education was ranting about in his latest outpouring of concern about the state of physical culture in North America, this seemed like a good point to briefly and succinctly review past human history in this regard. Hence Part V tackled that subject by answering the question: "What happened with sport and related physical activity historically? The discussion traced these activities briefly from primitive and preliterate societies to the present. *My effort to achieve historical perspective resulted in the belief that (1) an uneasy amalgam" forged from the past exists insofar as children, young adults, adults, senior, be they normal, accelerated, or special-needs people; and (2) physical activity education and related health information in advanced societies has been treated grossly inadequately and insufficiently as a subject of lesser importance in the education curriculum.*

To many people what I have to say here will probably mark me as a "mean old man and a spoilsport," a grinch trying to "upset the prevailing applecart…! However, the past few months have absolutely convinced me that we in the developed (?) world have our priorities all screwed up in relation to competitive sport and physical activity education. Frankly, I am so sick of "gold–medals this" and "own–the–podium that" that I feel completely frustrated by the money, time, and attention devoted to these activities for the "minute few"! Then, on top of the Olympics Games, we also have the Paralympic Games and the Special Olympics. (Fortunately, the latter two are more like what the "big one" ought to be!) All in all, however, enuf already…

*Please don't misunderstand me. I believe physical activity education and educational/recreational sport competition are wonderful activities for **all** people of all ages and conditions throughout their lives. There is evidence that such activity will enable people to live more fully and also to live healthier lives longer! However, my fundamental point is that—for the good of humankind—we must build from the ground up with **all** people!* As matters stand now, we do a fair to poor to "nil" job of physical activity education with the *very* large majority of youth (and somewhat worse for the "girl component of the mix"). Yet, when it comes to a minute fraction of youth—"accelerated and special"—within both education and the private sector, we actually do quite well to excellent to superb with competitive sport.

Why Should Competitive Sport Be Unique?

Think about it! Suppose we managed our affairs in this way with any other important subject or activity in the educational curriculum (e.g., English, science, math…)? The outcry would be so loud that all activity in our everyday world would be brought to a shrieking halt peremptorily. "How dare you deny this essential experience to my son (or daughter)? He (She) has

217

a right to the same advantages that all others get! Throw the legislators, the educators, and/or any other 'bum' responsible for this dereliction of duty out of office on his/her rump this very day!"

I simply can't understand why you, as intelligent people, can't see that somehow "going West" the cart has been put in front of the horse! Unless your son and daughter is gifted in regard to his/her heritage of physical skill, he/she is a *nonentity* in education being deprived of what could be–if properly stressed and taught–a truly important "physical educational experience". Such an experience would not only help him or her to learn better, but it would also help to keep this young person healthy now and prepare him/her attitude-wise and literally "movement-wise" for "the long journey ahead" through life.

Just consider the prevailing situation starkly! The folks promoting the present "upside-down" approach to their version of physical activity education, including "varsity sport" competition, for *all* youth will tell you that the present overemphasis for the few is *the* way to do it. Those "on the bottom," they say blithely, will be inspired by seeing "all these medals arriving on our shores". They will start working to "get there" too. I say: "Baloney"! These "physical klutzes"–as they see it–will never have a chance if affairs continue as they occur–or don't take place!–today. This will continue to be the case until –the next thing you know–these "people in control" today will convince politicians to still further arrange things the way they are in China. "What's this?", you say. The answer is to test little boys and girls for inherent physical ability early; take them from their parents; and send them to specially designed schools for early training. Then watch them "get those gold medals on 'the podium that their country owns'"! Wow! Glorioski! Eureka! Nirvana!

> Note: To me the logic of my above argument seems
> impeccable. The illogical response appears to be: 'Em that
> has, gits'. "That's the way the world is."

The Sport Hero Phenomenon

Following directly up on the "analysis of status" in Part IV of the role of competitive sport in North America as opposed to the what is (or isn't) happening with physical activity education (including recreational sport), I decided to include in Part V an historical summary of sport and related physical activity dating back to "Day #1" in human history.

Then in Part VI, I next felt it necessary to take my analysis of the existing, unfair, lopsided situation that exists one step further. Interestingly, and somewhat understandably but disgustingly, we now have what can be termed "The Sport Hero Phenomenon". As I see it, if you think there is merit to my argument about the inequality that exists in so-called democratic society with regard to overly emphasized competitive sport for a small minority as over against sound physical activity education for the large majority of the populace, you may also agree with my analysis of a developing situation that exists very largely for select males of the species.

History has been replete with the exploits of heroes, but has recorded relatively few of such achievements by heroines. It could be argued that today a society needs its heroes and its heroines as part of its growth and development process, as well as its pattern– maintenance process. If these leaders don't appear in the normal (abnormal?) course of events, it could be hypothesized further that society will somehow create them in sometimes unexpected places as they fulfill unusual roles. (Keep in mind that *a hero has "ability admired for his [or her] brave deeds and qualities."*)

A so-called *culture* hero appears to be a notch higher on the scale, however, and is explained as "*a mythicized historical figure who embodies the aspirations or ideals of a society.*" Certain, quite specific societal conditions provide greater opportunity for the individual with heroic qualities to emerge (e.g., war, emergencies, crises). Nevertheless, we might agree that such a person might appear at any time or place if several conditions prevail in any of life's recognized activities.

In the realm of sport, there were those who asserted that "we have seen the last of the athletic hero" (e.g., London, 1978). Yet, if society *needs* heroes, and if they are still emerging in ongoing societal life, is that not reason enough to believe that a true hero could conceivably emerge in competitive sport as well as in other activities? Admittedly, the right (i.e., correct or appropriate) conditions would have to be present (in some sequential order?) for the creation or establishment of such a person.

However, people need to understand what actually has happened through use of their own rational powers. Those people in organizations that are exploiting sport are increasingly luring a gullible public through clever marketed daily by into reactions dominated more by emotions than reason. It may well be necessary to reinforce "civic ego" at the various geographical levels (i.e. community, region, state or province, nation) by the creation of heroes and heroines in the various aspects of social living (including sport). However, the extent to which this should be done through the artificial creation of "dubious superheroes" is debatable. Question: Should society create such status for some even when such individuals do not appear normally in the course of ongoing events?

Should a Country Support the Olympic Games?

There's a vocal minority who believe the Olympic Games should be abolished. There's another minority, including the Games officials and the athletes, who obviously feel the enterprise is doing just fine. *In addition, there's a larger minority undoubtedly solidly behind the commercial aspects of the undertaking.* They have a good thing going; they like the Games the way they are developing— the bigger, the better! Finally, there's the vast majority to whom the Olympics are either interesting, somewhat interesting, or a bore. This "vast majority," if the Games weren't "there!" every four years, would probably agree that the world would go on just the same, and some other social phenomenon would take up their leisure time of those who watch this activity.

You will recall that I asked whether a country should be involved with, or continue involvement with, the ongoing Olympic Movement—as well as all highly competitive, professional sport—unless the people in that country first answer some basic questions. These questions ask to what extent such involvement can be related to the social and individual values that the country holds as important for all of its citizens. At present we do not know positively whether sport competition at either or all of the three levels (i.e., amateur, semi-professional, and professional) does indeed provide positive social and individual value (i.e., more value than disvalue) in the country concerned.

The answer to this problem should be determined as soon as possible through careful scientific assessment through the efforts of qualified social scientists and philosophers. We also need to asses the populace's opinions and basic beliefs about such involvement after the evidence becomes available!. If participation in competitive sport at each of the three levels can make this claim to being a social institution that provides positive value to the country, these efforts should be supported to the extent possible—including the sending of a team to future Olympic Games. *However, if sufficient funding for the support of all three levels of participation is simply not available, from either governmental or private sources, the expressed will of the people should be established to determine what priorities will be invoked after the evidence has been received and assessed by the public.*

Where Should We Want To Be?

Next, in Part VIII, I sought to make the case that sound physical activity education including an *intramural* competitive sport experience is good for all boys and girls as they grow up to adult status. I explained the need to monitor the growth and development pattern of the child. I argued that boys and girls today are simply not rugged enough, that a majority of them are either obese or overweight, and that they are mistakenly being allowed to lead "soft and easy" lives. Although parents should be careful not to employ undue pressures to influence the young person, nevertheless the child's basic needs must be met if a desirable result is anticipated.

However, it should be understood that there is much more to life than sport. Some people seem to think that a normal, healthy youngster should be playing tiddlywinks most of the time, while at the other extreme people go so far as to encourage regional and national sport tournaments for elementary school boys and girls. Some people even have elementary school children running the marathon! It is simply not possible to discuss organized sport for children and youth intelligently unless we are fully aware of the entire pattern of child growth and development. For example, what is the physical growth and developmental pattern of a ten-year old? What are the characteristics of this age? Or to put it another way, what are his or her needs? My recommendation here is that parents should answer some fundamental questions for themselves.

Questions Parents Should Ask

What questions should any parent ask? The answers—and I have arranged such questions in a sequential order that can be useful—is that there are a number of them as follows:

> 1. What Are My Child's Needs With Regard to
>   Physical Activity Education (including Sport)

First off, we should proceed on the assumption that a parent must strive to meet a child's basic needs. Thus, keeping that in mind, we must learn what excellent, good, fair, and indifferent physical development is. For example, we are told that boys and girls are not rugged enough today. We are told, also, that children are typically too fat. So we need to know what children and youth are getting today in elementary and secondary physical activity and related health and safety education.

2. How Do I Know That My Child/Youth Is Receiving a Fine Experience?

Then we need to know if this is enough. Does this concur for what I as a parent want for my child or young person? What sort of an "environment" is being provided? Are there any undue pressures? Under what conditions does competitive sport offer an ideal setting for teaching and learning? For example, will my child be introduced to contact/collision sport before maturity? Also, is he/she specializing unduly at too early an age?

Further, despite the fact that we want to guarantee the best type of sport and physical activity education for youth, we need to keep in mind that there is ever so much more to life than sport competition. So what we need in the final analysis is an educational environment that is best for children and youth in an ever-changing, complex, challenging world.

At this point let us be optimistic and prospective about this important matter. Accordingly, I would like to offer a "formula" that could well be tried out in communities of all sizes-and indeed is functioning in enlightened centers already. What I am recommending is steadily increasing cooperation between the recreation director and the physical activity educator/coach already. Basically, we know that boys and girls from eight to, say, 13 years of age are an interesting and challenging group with which to work. They are typically eager and anxious to try almost everything and anything. They respond readily to suggestion, and it makes us happy to see them at play (and occasionally "at work" too!). This is the age group where *all* children should *really* receive the finest of experiences!

As parents and enlightened citizens, we should encourage recreation directors to work more closely with school principals, the physical activity education supervisors (if your community is fortunate enough to have such people), and the high school physical activity educators and coaches. You may say that your community is already doing this to a degree. My response is **"To What Degree?"** Nevertheless, I'll wager that not many communities have come up with this idea. Why not encourage the high school physical activity education men and women teacher/coaches to suggest "amateur coaches" for your teams from a leaders corps they might recommend? These would be young coaches of both sexes who would receive planned recognition and small honoraria for devoted, capable assistance. These young people might even join the education profession eventually.

Here, I feel, is our greatest potential for coaching leadership. I am certain that in most communities we are not making the best use of such an excellent source for young, interested leadership. Incidentally, along the way we could be running clinics for these young people to develop their leadership potential even further. Also, most of these young people are going to stay right in your community, and it would be useful to them and the community to encourage this idea of community service through an internship experience. Some of them might even go on to follow this type of endeavor as a profession.

A Final Word

I believe physical activity education and educational/recreational sport competition are wonderful activities for **all** *people of all ages and conditions throughout their lives. There is evidence that such activity will enable people to live more fully and also to live healthier lives longer! However, my fundamental point is that—for the good—* **and the future!** *— of humankind—we must build from the ground up with* **all** *people!*

As matters stand now, we do a fair to poor to "nil" job of physical activity education with the *very* large majority of youth (and somewhat worse for the "girl component of the mix"). Yet, when it comes to a minute fraction of youth—"accelerated and special"—within both education and the private sector, we actually do quite well to excellent to superb with competitive sport.

Human physical activity, broadly interpreted and experienced under wise educational or recreational conditions, can indeed provide value and be a worthwhile social institution contributing vitally to the well being, ongoing health, and longevity of humankind?

References and Bibliography

Aburdene, P. & Naisbitt, J. (1992). *Megatrends for women*. NY: Villard Books. 388 p.

Adams, G.B. (1922) *Civilization during the Middle Ages*. NY: Charles Scribner's Sons.

Amara, R. (1981). The futures field. The Futurist, February.

American Alliance for Health, Physical Education, and Recreation (Spring 1957) Statement of policies and procedures for girls' and women's sport. *JOHPER*, 28, 6:57-58.

American Alliance for Health, Physical Education, Recreation and Dance (1962) *Professional preparation in health education, physical education, recreation education. Report of national conference*. Washington, DC: Author.

American Alliance for Health, Physical Education, Recreation and Dance. (1974). *Professional preparation in dance, physical education, recreation education, safety education, and school health education*. Report on national conference. Washington, DC: Author.

Anderson, W. T. (1996). *The Fontana postmodernism reader*, London: Fontana Press.

Anderson, W.T. (1997). *The future of the self: Inventing the postmodern person*. NY: Tarcher/Putnam.

Aronowitz, S. & Giroux, H.A. (1991). *Postmodern education: Politics, culture, and social criticsm*. Minneapolis, Univ. of Minnesota press.

Artz, F.B. (1981). *The mind of the Middle Ages*. (3rd Ed.). Chicago: Univ. of Chicago Press.

Asimov, I. (1970). The fourth revolution. *Saturday Review*. Oct. 24, 17-20.

Ayer, A. J. (1984) *Philosophy in the twentieth century*. NY: Vintahe.

Bagley, J.J. (1961). *Life in medieval England*. London: B.T. Batsford.

Ballou, R.B. (1965). *An analysis of the writings of selected church fathers to A.D. 394 to reveal attitudes regarding physical activity*. Doctoral dissertation, University of Oregon.

Barber, R. (1975). *The knight and chivalry*. Totowa, NJ: Rowman and Littlefield.

Barker, J. (1986). *The tournament in England, 1100-1400*. Suffolk: Boydell and Brewer.

Barney, R.K. (1985). The hailed, the haloed, and the hallowed: Sport heroes and their qualities—An analysis and hypothetical model for their commemoration. In *Sport History Official Report, Olympic Scientific Congress* (N. Mueller & J. Ruehl, eds.). Niederhausen, FRG: Schors Verlag.

Barrett, W. (1959). *Irrational man: A study in existential philosophy*. Garden City, NY: Doubleday.

Barzun, J. (1974). <u>The use and abuse of art</u>. Princeton: Princeton Univ. Press.

Bazzano, C. (1973). *The contribution of the Italian Renaissance to physical education*. Doctoral dissertation, Boston University.

Beeler, J. (1966). *Warfare in England*. Ithaca, NY: Cornell University Press.

Bennett, B.L. (1962). Religion and physical education. Paper presented at the Cincinnati Convention of the AAHPER, April 10.

Bentley, E. (1969). *The cult of the superman*. MA: Gloucester.

Bereday, G.Z.F. (1964). *Comparative method in education* (see pp. 11-27). New York: Holt, Rinehart and Winston.

Bereday, G.Z.F. (1969). Reflections on comparative methodology in education, 1964-1966. In M.A. Eckstein & H.J. Noah (Eds.), *Scientific investigations in comparative education* (pp. 3-24). New York: Macmillan.

Berelson, B. and Steiner, G. A. (1964). *Human Behavior*. NY: Harcourt, Brace, Jovanovich.

Berman, M. (2001) *The twilight of American culture*. NY: W.W. Norton.

Bury, J.B. (1955). *The idea of progress*. New York: Dover.

Bishop, G. *A $60 Million Dollar Palace for Texas High School Football The New York Times.Sports. Jan. 20, 2011*

Blinde, E.M. & McCallister, S.G. (1999). Women, disability, and sport and physical fitness activity: The intersection of gender and disability dynamics. *Research Quarterly for Sport and Exercise*, 70, 3, 303-312.

Bookwalter, K.W., & Bookwalter, C.W. (1980). *A review of thirty years of selected research on undergraduate professional preparation physical education programs in the United States*. Unionville, IN: Author.

Booth, F.W., & Chakravarthy, M.V. (2002). Cost and consequences of sedentary living: New battleground for an old enemy. *Research Digest (PCPFS)*, 3, 16, 1-8.

Borgman, A. (1993) *Crossing the postmodern divide*. Chicago: The
  University of Chicago Press.

Boorstin, D.J. (1961*). The image: Or what happened to the American
  dream*. London: Weidenfeld and Nicolson

Bottomley, F. (1979). *Attitudes toward the body in Western
  Christendom*. London: Lepus.

Bradbury, J. (1985). *The medieval archer*. NY: St. Martin's Press.

Broekhoff, J. ((1973). Chivalric education in the Middle Ages. In E. F.
  Zeigler, Ed. & Au.), *A history of sport and physical education
  to 1900* (pp. 225-234). Champaign, IL: Stipes.

Bronowski, J. & Mazlish, B. (1975). *The Western intellectual tradition:
  From Leonardo to Hegel*. New York: Harper & Row,

Broom, E., Clumpner, R., Pendleton, B., & Pooley, C. (Eds.), *Comparative
  physical education and sport*, Volume 5. Champaign, IL: Human Kinetics.

Broudy, H.S. (1961). *Building a philosophy of education*. 2nd ed.
  Englewood Cliffs, NJ: Prentice-Hall.

Brubacher, J. S. (1966). *A history of the problems of education*.
  (2nd Ed.). NY: McGraw-Hill.

Brubacher, J. S. (1969). *Modern philosophies of education* (4th ed.).
  New York: McGraw-Hill.

Bury, J. B. (1955). *The idea of progress*. New York: Dover.

Butler, J. D. (1957) *Four philosophies*. (Rev. Ed.). NY: Harper.

Butts, R. F. (1947). *A cultural history of education*. New York: McGraw-
  Hill.

Calin, W. (1966). *The epic quest*. Baltimore: Johns Hopkins Press.

Carlyle, T. (n.d.). *Heroes, hero worship and the heroic in history*. NY: A. L. Burt.

Carter, J.M. (May 1980). *Sport in the Bayeux Tapestry*, Canadian
  Journal of Sport History, XI, 1: 36-60.

Carter, J.M. (1981). *Ludi medi aevi: Studies in the history of
  medieval sport*. Manhattan, KS: Military Affairs Publishing.

Carter, J.M. (1988). *Sports and pastimes of the Middle Ages*. Lanham,
  MD: University Press of America.

Carter, J.M. (1992).*Medieval games; Sports and recreations in feudal
  society*. Westport, CT: Greenwood.

Castiglione, B. (1959). *The book of the courtier* (C.S. Singleton,
  trans.). NY: Doubleday.

Caxton, W. (1926). *The book of the order of chyvalry*. In A.T.
  Bayles, (Ed.). London: Oxford University Press.

Champion, S.G. & Short, D. (1951). *Readings from the world religions*.

Boston: Beacon.

Chaucer, G. (1991). *The Canterbury tales*. (Begun in 1387). NY: QPBC.

Childs, J.L. (1931). *Education and the philosophy of experimentalism*. NY: Appleton-Century-Crofts.

Clephan, C.R. (1919). *The tournament: Its periods and phases*. NY: Ungar.(Clepham, R.C.??)

Columbia Encyclopedia, The New (W.H. Harvey & J.S. Levey, Eds.). (1975). NY: Columbia University Press.

Commager, H.S. (1961). A quarter century—Its advances. *Look*, 25, 10 (June 6), 80-91.

Commission on Tests, College Entrance Examination Board. (Nov. 2, 1970). *The New York Times*.

Conant, J.B. (1963). *The education of American teachers* (pp. 122-123). New York: McGraw-Hill.

Contributions of physical activity to human well-being. (May, 1960) *Research Quarterly*, 31, 2 (Part II):261-375.

Cornish, F.W. (1901). *Chivalry*. NY: Macmillan.

Cosentino, F. & Howell, M.L. (1971). *A history of physical education in Canada*. Don Mills, Ont.: General Publishing Co.

Coulton, G.G. (1960). Medieval village, manor and monastery. NY: Harper.

Cowell, C.C. (1960). The contributions of physical activity to social development. *Research Quarterly*, 31, 2 (May, Part II), 286-306.

Crepeau, R. Personal e-mail correspondence. 2011/01/20.

Cryderman, K. (2001). Sport's culture of adultery. *The Vancouver Sun* (Canada), August 21, C5.

Crossland, J. (1956). *Medieval French literature*. Oxford: Basil Blackwell.

Cuff, J.H. (1983). Just regular guys. *The Globe and Mail* (Toronto), August 20, 3.

Cummins, J. *The hound and the hawk: The art of medieval hunting*. NY: St. Martin's Press.

Czikszentmihalyi, M. (1993). *The evolving self: A psychology for the third millenium*. NY: Harper Perennial.

DeMott, B. (1969). How existential can you get? *The New York Times Magazine*, March 23, pp. 4, 6, 12, 14.

Depauw, K.P. (1997). The (in)visibility of disability: Cultural contexts and "sporting bodies," *Quest*, 49, 416-430

Dewey, J. (1938). *Logic, the theory of inquiry*. NY: Holt, Rinehart and Winston.

Dubin, R. (1978) *Theory building*. NY: The Free Press.

Durant, W. (1938). The story of philosophy. (New rev. ed.). NY: Garden City.

Durant, W. (1950). *The age of faith*. NY: Simon and Schuster.

Durant, W. & Durant, A. (1968). *The lessons of history*. New York: Dover.

Elliott, R. (1927). *The organization of professional training in physical education in state universities*. New York: Columbia Teachers College.

Encarta World English Dictionary, The. (1999). NY: St. Martin's Press.

Encyclopedia of Philosophy, The (P. Edwards, Ed.). (1967). (8 vols.). NY: Macmillan & Free Press.

English, E. (1984). Sport, the blessed medicine of the Renaissance. In *Proceedings of the North American Society for the Study of Sport History* (D. Wiggins, Ed.). Kansas State University Press, Manhattan.

Eyler, M.H. (1956). *Origins of some modern sports*. Ph.D. dissertation, University of Illinois, Champaign-Urbana.

Fairs, J. R. (1973). The influence of Plato and Platonism on the development of physical education in Western culture. In E. F. Zeigler (Ed. & Au.), *A history of sport and physical education to 1900*, pp. 155-166 Champaign, IL: Stipes.

Feibleman, J. (1973). *Understanding philosophy*. NY: Dell.

Feschuk, S. (2002). Night of the Olympic dead. *National Post* (Canada), Feb. 16, B10.

Finley, M.I. (1965) *The world of Odysseus*. NY: Viking.

Fishwick, M. (1969). *The hero, American style*. NY: David McKay

Flach, J. (1904). Chivalry. In *Medieval civilization* (D. Munro & G. Sellery, Eds.). NY: Century.

Flath, A.W. (1964). *A history of relations between the National Collegiate Athletic Association and the Amateur Athletic Union of the United States (1905-1963)*. Champaign, IL: Stipes.

Forsyth, I.H. (April 1978). The theme of cockfighting in Burgundian Romanesque sculpture. *Speculum*: 252-282.

Fraleigh, W.P. (1970). Theory and design of philosophic research in physical education. *Proceedings of the National College Physical*

Education Association for Men, Portland, OR, Dec. 28.

Froissart, J. (1842). *Chronicles of England, France, Spain, and the adjoining countries*. (2 Vols.). (T. Johnes, trans.). London: Smith.

Gautier, L. (1989). *Chivalry*. London: Bracken. (This book was originally published as *La Chevalrie* in 1883 in Paris.)

Geiger, G.R. (1955). An experimentalistic approach to education. In N.B. Henry (Ed.), *Modern philosophies and education* (Part I). Chicago: Univ. of Chicago Press.

Gies, F. (1964). *The knight in history*. NY: Harper & Row.

Gimpel, J. (1976). *The medieval machine: The industrial revolution of the Middle Ages*. NY; Holt, Rinehart and Winston.

Glasser, W. (1972). *The identity society*. NY: Harper & Row.

Glassford, R.G. (1970) *Application of a theory of games to the transitional Eskimo culture*. Ph.D. dissertation, University of Illinois, Urbana.

Good, C.F., & Scates, D.E. (1954). *Methods of research* New York: Appleton-Century-Crofts.

Green. H. (1986). *Fit for America*. Baltimore: The Johns Hopkins University Press..

Greene, T.M. (1955). A liberal Christian idealist philosophy of education. In N.B. Henry (Ed.), *Modern Philosophies of education*. Chicago, Univ. of Chicago Press.

Guttman, A. (1986). *Sports spectators*. NY: Columbia University Press.

Hahm, C. H., Beller, J .M., & Stoll, S. K. (1989). *The Hahm-Beller Values Choice Inventory*. Moscow, Idaho: Center for Ethics, The University of Idaho.

Handlin, O. et al. (1967). Harvard guide to American history. NY: Atheneum

Haskins, C. H. (1995). *The Normans in European history*. NY: Barnes & Noble.

Hayes, C. (1961). *Nationalism: A religion*. New York: Macmillan.

Heilbroner, R.L. (1960). *The future as history*. New York: Harper & Row.

Heinemann, F.H. (1958). *Existentialism and the modern predicament*. NY: Harper & Row.

Henricks, T.S. (1982). Sport and social hierarchy in medieval England. *Journal of Sport History*, IX, 2: 20-37.

Henricks, T.S. (1991) *Disputed pleasures: Sport and society in pre-*

industrial England. Westport, CT: Greenwood.

Henry, J. (1963). *Culture against man.* NY: Random House

Hershkovits, M.J. (1955). *Cultural anthropology.* New York: Knopf.

Hess, F.A. (1959). *American objectives of physical education from 1900 to 1957 assessed in light of certain historical events.* Ph.D. dissertation, New York University.

Hocking, W.E. (1928). *The meaning of God in human experience.* New Haven, CT: Yale University Press.

Hoernle, R. F. A. (1927). *Idealism as a philosophy.* NY: Doubleday.

Holmes, U.T. *Daily living in the twelfth century* Madison, WI: Univ. of Wisconsin Press.

Homer. (1951). *The Iliad* (R. Lattimore, trans.). Chicago: Univ. of Chicago Press.

Homer. (1950). *The Odyssey* (S.H. Butcher & A. Lang, trans.). NY: The Modern Library.

Homer-Dixon, T. (2001). *The ingenuity gap.* Toronto: Vintage Canada.

Hook, S. (1955). *The hero in history.* Boston: Beacon Press.

Horne, H.H. (1942). An idealistic philosophy of education. In *Proceedings of the National Society for the Study of Education,* Part I (Forty-First Yearbook), N.B.Henry (Ed.). Chicago, IL: University of Chicago Press, pp. 139-196.

Huizinga, J. (1954). *The waning of the Middle Ages.* NY: Doubleday-Anchor.

Huntington, S. P. (June 6, 1993). World politics entering a new phase, *The New York Times,* E19

Huntington, S. P. (1998). *The Clash of Civilizations (and the Remaking of World Order.* NY: Touchstone.

Huxley, J. (1957). *New wine for new bottles.* NY: Harper & Row.

Jaeger, W.W. (1939). *Paideia: The ideals of Greek culture.* NY: Oxford University Press.

James, W. (1929). *Varieties of religious experience.* NY: Longmans, Green.

Jameson, F. (1992). Postmodernism. Durham, NC: Duke University Press.

Johnson, H.M. (1969). The relevance of the theory of action to historians. *Social Science Quarterly,* 2: 46-58.

Johnson, H. M. (1994). Modern organizations in the Parsonsian theory of action. In A. Farazmond, *Modern organizations: Administrative theory in contemporary society,* pp. 57 et ff. Westport, CT: Praeger.

Joseph, L.M. (1949). *Gymnastics: From the Middle Ages to the 18th century.* CIBA Symposium, 10, 5: 1030-1060.

Kahn, R. (1958). Money-muscles—and myths. In *Mass leisure* (E. Larrabee & R. Meyersohn, Eds.). Glencoe, IL: The Free Press.

Kaplan, A. (1961). *The new world of philosophy.* Boston: Houghton Mifflin.

Kateb, G. (Spring, 1965) Utopia and the good life. *Daedulus,* 92, 2:455-472.

Kaufmann, Walter. (1976). *Religions in four dimensions.* NY: Reader's Digest Press.

Kavussanu, M. & Roberts, G.C. (2001). Moral functioning in sport: An achievement goal perspective. *Journal of Sport and Exercise Psychology,* 23, 37-54

Keen, M. (1984). *Chivalry.* New Haven: Yale University Press.

Kennedy, J. F. (1958). (From an address by him in Detroit, Michigan while he was a U.S. Senator.)

Kennedy, P. (1987). *The rise and fall of the great powers.* NY: Random House.

Kennedy, P. (1993). *Preparing for the twenty-first century.* New York: Random House.

Kilgour, R.L. (1966). *The decline of chivalry.* Gloucester, MA: Smith.

Klapp. O.E. (1972). *Heroes, villains and fools: Reflections of the American character.* San Diego, CA: Aegis.

Kneller, G.F. (1984). *Movements of thought in modern education.* New York: John Wiley & Sons.

Krikorian, Y. H. (1944). *Naturalism and the human spirit.* NY: Columbia University Press.

Lacroix, P. (1974). *Military and religious life in the Middle Ages and at the period of the Renaissance.* London: Chapman & Hall.

Lauwerys, J. A. (1959) *The philosophical approach to comparative education.* International Review of Education, V, 283-290.

LeGoff, J. (1980). *Time, work and culture in the Middle Ages.* Chicago: Univ. of Chicago Press.

Lenk, H. (1994). Values changes and the achieving society: A sociol-philosophical perspective. In *Organization for economic co-operation and development, OECD Societies in Transition.* (pp. 81-94)

Leonard, F. E., & Affleck G. B. (1947). *The history of physical education* (3rd ed.). Philadelphia: Lea & Febiger.

Lipset. S. M. (1973). National character. In D. Koulack & D. Perlman (Eds.), *Readings in social psychology: Focus on Canada.* Toronto: Wiley.

London, H. (1978). The vanishing athletic hero, or whatever happened to sacrifice? Sport section, *The New York Times*, April 23, 2.

Long, W. (2001. Athletes losing faith in hard work. *The Vancouver Sun* (Canada), Jan. 31. E5.

Lubin, H. (1968). The adventurer-warrior hero. In *Heroes and anti-heroes* (H. Lubin, Ed.). San Francisco: Chandler.

Lumpkin, A., Stoll, S.K., & Beller, J.M. (1999). *Sport ethics: Applications for fair play* (2nd Ed.). St. Louis: McGraw-Hill.

MacIntyre, A. (1967). Existentialism. In P. Edwards, ed., *The Encyclopedia of Philosophy*. Vol. 3, NY: Macmillan

Magill, F.N. & Staff. (1961). *Masterworks of world philosophy*. NY: Harper & Row.

Malina, R. M. (2001). Tracking of physical activity across the lifespan. *Research Digest (PCPFS)*, 3-14, 1-8.

Marrou, H. I. (1964). *A history of education in antiquity*. Trans. George Lamb. New York: New American Library.

Marx, L. (1990). Does improved technology mean progress? In Teich, A. H. (Ed.), *Technology and the future*. NY: St. Martin's Press

Matthew, D. (1983). *Atlas of Medieval Europe*. NY: Facts on File.

McCurdy, J.H. (1901). Physical training as a profession. *American Physical Education Review*, 6, 4:311-312.

McGowan, J. (1991). *Postmodernism and its critics*. Ithaca: Cornell University Press.

McIntosh, P. C. (1957). "Physical education in Renaissance Italy and Tudor England." In *Landmarks in the history of physical education* (J. G. Dixon, P. C. McIntosh, A. D. Munrow, & R. F. Willetts). London: Routledge & Kegan Paul.

McLean, T. (1984). *The English at play in the Middle Ages*. England: Windsor Forest. ???

McNeill W. H. (1963). *The rise of the West*. Chicago: Univ. of Chicago Press.

Meller, W. C.) (1924). *A knight's life in the days of chivalry*. London: T. Werner Lowrie.

Melnick, R. (1984). *Visions of the future*. Croton-on-Hudson, NY: Hudson Institute.

Mergen, F.. (1970). Man and his environment. *Yale Alumni*

Magazine, XXXIII, 8 (May), 36-37.

Mills, C. (1826). *The history of chivalry*. Philadelphia: Carey & Lea.

Mitchell, R. J. & Leys, M. D. R. (1950). *A history of the English people*. Toronto: Longmans Green.

Monckton, O. P. (1913). *Pastimes in times past*. Philadelphia: J. P. Lippincott.

Moolenijzer, N. J. (1973). The legacy from the Middle Ages. In E. F. Zeigler, E. F. (Ed. & Au.), *A history of sport to 1900*. Champaign, IL: Stipes.

Morford, W. R. & S.. J. Clark. (1976). The agon motif. In *Exercise and Sports Sciences Reviews* (Vol. 4). Santa Barbara, CA: Journal Publishing Associates, pp. 163-193.

Morgan, K. O. (Ed.). (1988). *Oxford history of Britain*, The. NY: Oxford

Morris, V. C. (1956). Physical education and the philosophy of education. *Journal of Health, Physical Education and Recreation*, (March), 21-22, 30-31.

Morrow, L. D. (1975). *Selected topics in the history of physical education in Ontario: From Dr. Egerton Ryerson to the Strathcona Trust (1844-1939)*. Ph.D. dissertation, The University of Alberta.

Muller, H. J. (1952). The uses of the past: Profiles of former societies. NY: Oxford University Press.

Muller, H. J. (1963). *The uses of the past*. NY: New American Library.

Muller, H. J. (1961). *Freedom in the ancient world*.

Muller, H. J. (1963). *Freedom in the Western world*. NY: Harper & Row.

Murray, B. G. Jr. (1972). What the ecologists can teach the economists. *The New York Times Magazine*, December 10, 38-39, 64-65, 70, 72.

Naipaul, V.S. (Oct 30, 1990). "Our Universal Civilization." The 1990 Winston Lecture, The Manhattan Institute, *New York Review of Books*, p. 20.

Naisbitt, J. (1982). *Megatrends*. New York: Warner.

Naisbitt, J. & Aburdene, P. (1990). *Megatrends* 2000. New York: Wm. Morrow.

National Geographic Society (M. Severy, Ed.). (1969). *The age of chivalry*. Washington, DC: National Geographic Society.

Naylor, D. (2002), In pursuit of level playing fields. *The Globe and Mail (Canada)*, March 9, S1.

Nevins, A. (1962). *The gateway to history*. Garden City, NY: Doubleday.

New York Times, The. (1970). Report by Commission on Tests of the

College Entrance Examination Board, Nov. 2.

Nickel, H. (1986). Games and pastimes. In J.R. Strayer (Ed.),
   Dictionary of the Middle Ages. NY: Scribner's. Pp.???

Nietzsche, F. (1958). *Thus spake Zarathustra*. (Transl. by A. Tille). London:
   J.M. Dent & Sons.

Norman, A.V.B. (1971). *The medieval soldier*. NY: Barnes & Noble.

Oldenbourgh, Z. (1948). *The world is not enough*. NY: Balantyne
   Books.

Olivova, V. From the arts of chivalry to gymnastics. *Canadian Journal
   of Sport History*, XII, 2: 29-55.

Olmert, M. (Fall 1984). Chaucer's little lotteries: The literary use of a
   medieval game. *Arete: Journal of Sport Literature* II, 1:171-182.

Olson, G. (1980). *Reading as recreation in the later Middle Ages*.
   Ithaca, NY: Cornell Univ. Press.

Oldenbourgh, Z. (1948). The world is not enough. NY: Balantyne
   Books.

Osterhoudt, R G. *Sport as a form of human fulfillment: An organic
   philosophy of sport history*. (Vol. I and II).Victoria, Canada: Trafford.

Painter, S. (1962). *French chivalry*. Baltimore: Johns Hopkins Press.

Paton, G.A. (1975). The historical background and present status of
   Canadian physical education. In E.F. Zeigler (Ed.), *A history of
   physical education and sport in the United States and Canada* (pp.
   441-443). Champaign, IL: Stipes.

Perry, R.B. (1955). *Present philosophical tendencies*. NY: George
   Braziller.

Platt, C. (1979). *The atlas of medieval man*. NY: St. Martin's Press.

Plumb, J.H. (1961). *Renaissance profiles*. NY: Harper & Row.

Priest, R.F., Krause, J.V., & Beach, J. (1999). Four-year changes in
   college athletes' ethical value choices in sports situations. *Research
   Quarterly for Exercise and Sport*, 70, 1, 170-178.

Province, The (Vancouver, Canada) (2000). Drug allegations
   rock sports world. July 3, A2.

Rajchman J. & West, C. (Eds.). (1985). *Post-analytic philosophy*. NY:
   Columbia Univ. Press.

Rand, A. (1960). *The romantic manifesto*. New York: World Publishing
   Co.

Random House dictionary of the English language (1967) (Jess Stein, Ed.). NY:

Random House.

Rees-Mogg, W. (1988). The decline of the Olympics into physical and moral squalor. *Coaching Focus*, 8 (1988),

Reisner, E.H. (1925). *Nationalism and education since 1789*. New York: Macmillan.

Renson, R. (1976). *The Flemish Archery Guilds: From defense mechanisms to sports institutions*. Mainz: Dokumente des V HISPA Kongresses, pp. 135-139.

Report on National Conference. Washington, DC: Author. Bennett, B.L. (1962). Religion and physical education. Paper presented at the Cincinnati Convention of the AAHPER, April 10.

Riesman, D. (1954). The themes of heroism and weakness in the structure of Freud's thought. In *Selected Essays from Individualism Reconsidered*. Garden City, NY: Doubleday.

Roberts, J. M. (1993). *A short history of the world*. NY: Oxford University Press.

Rorty, R. (1997) *Achieving our country*. Cambridge, MA: Harvard University Press

Rowling, M. (1968). *Everyday life in medieval times*. NY: Dorset.

Royce, J.R. (1964). Paths to knowledge. In *The encapsulated man*. Princeton, NJ: Van Nostrand.

Rudd, A., Stoll, S.K., & Beller, J.M. (1999). Measuring moral and social character among a group of Division 1A college athletes, non-athletes, and ROTC military students. *Research Quarterly for Exercise and Sport*, 70 (Suppl. 1), 127.

Rudorff, R. (1974). *Knights and the age of chivalry*. NY: Viking Press.

Russell, B. (1959). *Wisdom of the West*. London: Rathbone Books.

Sage, G.H. (1988, October). "Sports participation as a builder of character?" *The World and I*, 3, 629-641.

Scarre, C. (1993). *Smithsonian timelines of the ancient world*. London: Dorling Kindersly.

Schlesinger, A.M. (1998). (Rev. & Enl.).*The disuniting of America*. NY: W.W. Norton.

Schopenhauer, A. (1946). The world as will and idea. In F.N. Magill (Ed.), *Master-works of philosophy*. NY: Doubleday.

Schrodt. B. Sports of the Byzantine Empire, *The Journal of Sport History*, VIII, 3: 40-59.

Sellars, R.W. (1932). *The philosophy of physical realism*. NY:

Macmillan.

Sheldon, W. H. (with the collaboration of S. S. Stevens and W. B. Tucker). (1940). *The Varieties of Human Physique*. New York: Harper and Brothers.

Sheldon, W. H. (with the collaboration of S. S. Stevens). (1942). *The Varieties of Temperament*. New York: Harper and Brothers.

Sigerist, H.E. (1956). *Landmarks in the history of hygiene*. London: Oxford University Press.

Silvers, S. (1984). Letter to the Editor. *Sports Illustrated*, October 29.

Simpson, G.G. (1949). *The meaning of evolution*. New Haven & London: Yale University Press.

Skaset, H.B., Email correspondence. May 14, 2002.

Smith, H. (1831). *Festivals, games, and amusements*. London: Colburn & Bentley.

Sparks, W. (1992). Physical education for the 21st Century: Integration, not specialization. *NAPEHE: The Chronicle of Physical Education in Higher Education*, 4, 1:1-10-11.

Spears, B. & Swanson, R. (1988). *History of sport and physical education in the United States*. Dubuque, IA: Champaionship Books.

Spencer-Kraus, P. (1969). The application of "linguistic phenomenology" to the philosophy of physical education and sport. M.A. thesis, University of Illinois, U-C.

Spiegelberg, H. (1976). *The phenomenological movement: An introduction*. (Vol. 1, Rev. Ed.). The Hague: Nijhoff.

Spretnak, C. (1991). *States of grace: The recovery of meaning in the postmodern age*. NY: Harper/SanFrancisco.

Stark, S.D. (1987). Entertainment section, *The New York Times*, February 22, 19.

Stoll, S. K. & Beller, J. M. (1998). *Sport as education: On the edge*. NY: Columbia University Teachers College.

Steinhaus, A.H. (1952). Principal principles of physical education. In *Proceedings of the College Physical Education Association*. Washington, DC: AAHPER, pp. 5-11.

Strohmeyer, H. (1977). Physical education of the princes in the late Middle Ages as depicted by two works of the Styrian Abbot, Engelbert of Admont (1250-1331 A.D.). *Canadian Journal of Sport and Physical Education*, 1: 38-48.

Ten events that shook the world between 1984 and 1994. (Special Report). *Utne Reader*, 62 (March/April 1994): 58-74

Tibbetts, J. (2002). Spend more on popular sports, Canadians say, *National Post* (Canada), A8, April 15.

Tierney, B. (1974). *The Middle Ages, Vol. II: Readings in Medieval History.* (2nd Ed.). NY: Knopf.

Treharne, R.F. & Fullard, H. (Eds.). (1961). *Muir's New School Atlas of Universal History.* (21st Ed.). Barnes & Noble.

Tuchman, B.W. (1978). *A distant mirrow: The calamitous 14th century.* NY: Knopf.

Ten events that shook the world between 1984 and 1994. (Special Report). *Utne Reader,* 62 (March/April 1994):58-74.

Thomas, K. (Dec. 1964). Work and leisure in pre-industrial society. *Past and present,* 29: 50-62.

Tibbetts, J. (2002). Spend more on popular sports, Canadians say, *National Post* (Canada), A8, April 15.

Toffler, A. (1970). *Future shock.* New York: Random House.

Toffler, A. (1980). *The third wave.* New York: Bantam Books.

Toynbee, A.J. (1947). *A study of history.* NY: Oxford University Press.

Ueberhorst, H. (Ed.) (1978). *Geschichte der Leibesuebungen (*Vol. 2). Berlin: Verlag Bartels & Wernitz.

Ullman, W. (1965). *A history of political thought: The Middle Ages.* Baltimore, MD: Penguin.

Van Dalen, D.B. (1973). The idea of history of physical education during the Middle Ages and Renaissance. In E.F. Zeigler (Ed. & Au.), *A history of sport and physical education to 1900 (*pp. 217-224). Champaign, IL: Stipes.

Van Dalen, D.B., E.D. Mitchell, & B.L. Bennett. (1953). *A world history of physical education.* (1st Ed.). Englewood Cliffs, NJ: Prentice-Hall. (A second edition was also published.)

VanderZwaag, H.J. (1982). Background, meaning, and significance. In E. F. Zeigler, (Ed. & Au.). Physical education and sport: An Introduction (p. 54). Philadelphia: Lea & Febiger.

Veblen, T. (1899). *The theory of the leisure class.* NY: Macmillan.

Von Neumann, J. & Morgenstern, O. (1947). *The theory of games and economic behavior.* (2nd ed.). Princeton: Princeton University Press.

Wallis, D. (2002). Annals of Olympics filled with dubious decisions. *National Post* (Canada), Feb. 16, B2.

Warre-Cornish, F. (1901). *Chivalry.* London: Swan Sonnenschein.

Wecter, D. (1941). *The hero in America: A chronicle of hero worship*. NY: Charles
   Scribner's Sons.

Weiner, J. (Jan.-Feb. 2000). Why our obsession has ruined the game;
   and how we can save it. *Utne Reader*, 97, 48-50.

Weinstein, M. (1991). Critical thinking and the post-modern challenge
   to educational practice. *Inquiry: Critical Thinking Across the
   Disciplines*, 7:1, 1,14.

White, M. (1962). *The age of analysis*. Boston: Houghton Mifflin.

White, L. (1962). *Medieval technology and social change*. London:
   Oxford University Press.

Wilcox, R. C. (1991). Sport and national character: An empirical analysis.
   Journal of Comparative Physical Education and Sport., XIII(1), 3-27.

Wild, J. Education and human society: A realistic view. In N.B.
    Henry (Ed.), *Modern philosophies and education* (Part I).
    (1955). Chicago, Univ. of Chicago Press.

Williams, J. Paul. (1952). *What Americans believe and how they
   worship.* New York: Harper & Row.

Windelband, W. (1901). *A histoty of philosophy*. (Vol. I and II). (Rev.
   Ed.). NY: Harper & Row.

Wood, M. (1987). *In search of the Dark Ages*. NY: Facts on File.

Woodward, W. H. (1905). *Vittorino da Feltre and other humanist
   educators*. Cambridge University Press. (Reprinted from 1897 ed.).

Woody, T. (1949). *Life and education in early societies*. New York:
   Macmillan.

Zeigler, E. F. (April, 1948), Implications of the study of body types for
   physical education. *JOPERD, 15, 3:240-42, 254.*

Zeigler, E. F. (1951). *A history of undergraduate professional
   preparation in physical education in the United States, 1861-1948.*
   Eugene, OR: Oregon Microfiche

Zeigler, E. F. (1962). A history of professional preparation for physical
   education in the United States (1861-1961). In *Professional preparation in health
   education, physical education, and recreation education* (pp.116-133). Washington,
   DC: The American Association for Health, Physical Education, and
   Recreation.

Zeigler, E. F. (1964). *Philosophical foundations for physical, health, and
   recreation education*. Englewood Cliffs, NJ: Prentice-Hall.

Zeigler, E. F. (1965). *A brief introduction to the philosophy of religion.*
   Champaign, IL: Stipes.

Zeigler, E. F. (1968). *Problems in the history and philosophy of physical education and sport*. Englewood Cliffs, NJ: Prentice-Hall.

Zeigler, E. F. (Ed. & author). (1973). *A history of physical education and sport to 1900*. Champaign, IL: Stipes.

Zeigler, E. F. (1975). Historical perspective on contrasting philosophies of professional preparation for physical education in the United States. In *Personalizing physical education and sport philosophy* (pp. 325-347). Champaign, IL: Stipes.

Zeigler, E. F. (Ed. & author). (1975). *A history of physical education and sport in the United States and Canada*. Champaign, IL: Stipes.

Zeigler, E. F. (1977a). *Physical education and sport philosophy*. Englewood Cliffs, NJ: Prentice-Hall.

Zeigler, E. F. (1977b). Philosophical perspective on the future of physical education and sport. In R. Welsh (Ed.), *Physical education: A view toward the future* (pp. 36-61). Saint Louis: C.V. Mosby.

Zeigler, E. F. (1979). The past, present, and recommended future development in physical education and sport in North America. In *Proceedings of The American Academy of Physical Education* (G.M. Scott (Ed.), Washington, DC: The American Alliance for Health, Physical Education, Recreation, and Dance.

Zeigler, E. F. (1980). An evolving Canadian tradition in the new world of physical education and sport. In S.A. Davidson & P. Blackstock (Eds.), *The R. Tait McKenzie Addresses* (pp. 53-62). Ottawa, Canada: Canadian Association for Health, Physical Education and Recreation.

Zeigler, E. F. (1983a). Relating a proposed taxonomy of sport and developmental physical activity to a planned inventory of scientific findings. *Quest*, 35, 54-65.

Zeigler, E .F. (1986a). Undergraduate professional preparation in physical education, 1960-1985. *The Physical Educator*, 43 (1), 2-6.

Zeigler, E. F. (1986b). *Assessing sport and physical education: Diagnosis and projection*. Champaign, IL: Stipes.

Zeigler, E. F. (Spring, 1987). Babe Ruth or Lou Gehrig: A United States' dilemma. *The Physical Educator*, 44, 2:325-329.

Zeigler, E. F. *et al.* (1988a). *A history of physical education and sport*. Champaign, IL: Stipes.

Zeigler, E. F. (1988b). Physical education and sport in the Middle Ages. In E.F. Zeigler, (Ed. & Au.), *History of physical education and sport* (pp. 57-102). Champaign, IL: Stipes.

Zeigler, E. F. (1988c). A comparative analysis of undergraduate professional preparation in physical education in the United States and Canada. In

Zeigler, E. F. (1990). *Sport and physical education: Past, present, future*. Champaign,

IL: Stipes.

Zeigler, E. F. (May 1993). Chivalry's influence on sport and physical training in Medieval Europe. *Canadian Journal of History of Sport*, XXIV, 1:1-17.

Zeigler, E. F. (1994a) *Critical Thinking for the Professions: Health, Sport and Physical Education, Recreation, and Dance*. Champaign IL: Stipes Publishing L.L.C.

Zeigler, E. F. (ed. & au.). (1994b) *Physical education and kinesiology in North America: Professional and scholarly foundations*. Champaign, IL: Stipes Publishing Co.

Zeigler, E. F. (Sept.,1994c). Physical education's "principal principles". JOPERD, 54, 4-5. This was published, also, in the CAHPERD Journal, Spring, 1995, Vol. 61, No. 1, 20-21.

Zeigler, E.F. (1996). Historical perspective on "quality of life": Genes. memes, and physical activity. *Quest* , 48, 246-263.

Zeigler, E. F. (2003). *Socio-Cultural Foundations of Physical Education and Educational Sport*. Aachen, Germany: Meyer & Meyer Sport.

Zeigler, E. F. (2005). *History and Status of American Physical Education and Educational Sport*. Bloomington, IN: Trafford.

Zeigler, E. F. (Spring, 2006b) What the field of physical (activity) education should do in the immediate future," *The Journal of the International Council of Health, Physical Education, Recreation, Sport, and Dance*, XLII, 2:35-39. (This article was published in 2006 also in the *ICHPERSD Journal of Research in Health, Physical Education, Recreation, Sport, and Dance*.)

Zeigler, E. F. (2010). *Philosophy of Physical Activity Education (Including Educational Sport)*, p. 67. Victoria, BC: Trafford.

Zeigler, E. F. and Bowie, G. W. (1983). *Management competency development in physical education and sport*. Philadelphia: Lea & Febiger.

Zeldin, T. (1994). *An intimate history of humanity*. NY: HarperCollins.

Zetterberg, H.L. (1965). *On theory and verification in sociology*. Totowa, NJ: The Bedminster Press.